FXT

FUNCTIONAL
CROSS
TRAINING

THE REVOLUTIONARY, ROUTINE-BUSTING
APPROACH TO TOTAL-BODY FITNESS

BRETT STEWART & JASON WARNER

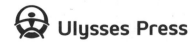
P9-DWD-691

 Ulysses Press

CALGARY PUBLIC LIBRARY

JUN - 2014

Text Copyright © 2014 Brett Stewart and Jason Warner. Design and concept © 2014 Ulysses Press and its licensors. All rights reserved. No part of this publication may be reproduced, stored in a retrieval system, or transmitted in any form or by any means (including but not limited to photocopying, electronic devices, digital versions, and the Internet) without the prior written permission of the publisher, nor be otherwise circulated in any form of binding or cover other than that in which it is published and without a similar condition being imposed on the subsequent purchaser.

Published in the United States by
Ulysses Press
P.O. Box 3440
Berkeley, CA 94703
www.ulyssespress.com

ISBN13: 978-1-61243-235-9
Library of Congress Control Number 2013938281

Printed in the United States by United Graphics, Inc.

10 9 8 7 6 5 4 3 2 1

Acquisitions Editor: Keith Riegert
Managing Editor: Claire Chun
Editor: Lily Chou
Proofreader: Lauren Harrison
Index: Sayre Van Young
Front cover design: what!design @ whatweb.com
Layout and production: Jake Flaherty
Cover photographs: rope climb © holbox/shutterstock.com; weight lifter © Pavel L Photo and Video/
    shutterstock.com; squat © Maridav/shutterstock.com
Interior photographs: see page 191
Models: Austin Akre, Brian Burns, Evan Clontz, Lewis Elliot, Mary J. Gines, Brett Stewart, Kristen
    Stewart, Chad Taylor

Distributed by Publishers Group West

Please Note: This book has been written and published strictly for informational purposes, and in no way should be used as a substitute for consultation with health care professionals. You should not consider educational material herein to be the practice of medicine or to replace consultation with a physician or other medical practitioner. The authors and publisher are providing you with information in this work so that you can have the knowledge and can choose, at your own risk, to act on that knowledge. The authors and publisher also urge all readers to be aware of their health status and to consult health care professionals before beginning any health program.

Contents

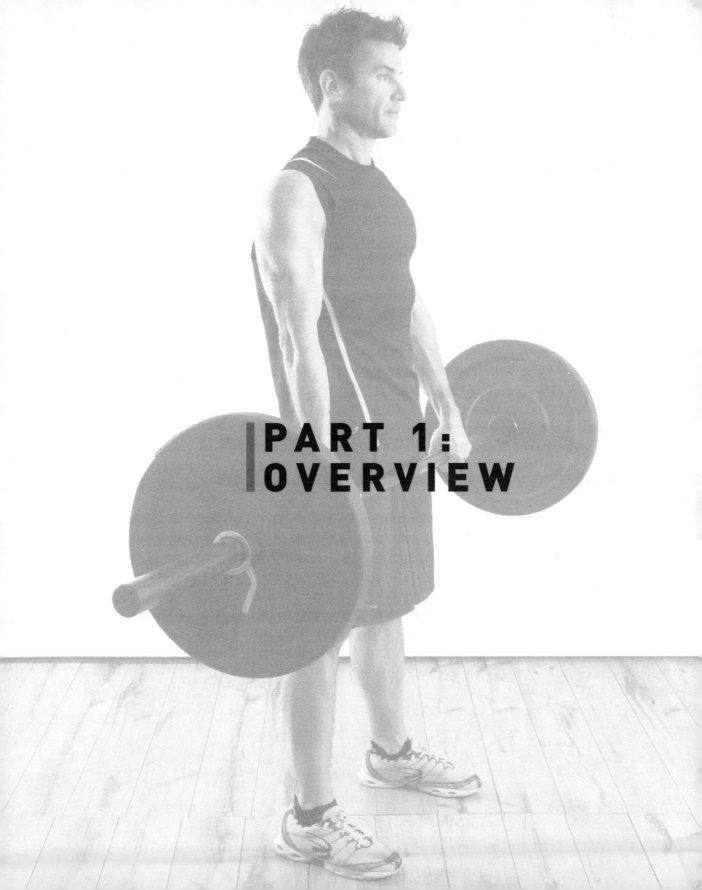

PART 1: OVERVIEW

Introduction

Embracing a spectrum of different workout methods, cross training is the best way to produce a fit, slender body while achieving peak overall fitness. *Functional Cross Training* is a step-by-step guide that brings together this wide range of cutting-edge techniques, including plyometrics, intense circuit training, weightlifting, and gym-free bodyweight exercises. The results are astounding—dramatically increased power, incredible endurance, packed-on lean muscle mass and greatly reduced body fat.

So? What does that really mean to you and your fitness? What makes functional cross training so revolutionary?

Functional cross training (or FXT) can—and will—change your life by modifying the way you look at fitness. Through years of research and testing, we developed a program that's easy to remember, simple to follow, and extremely effective for all individuals regardless of age, weight, current fitness level or lifestyle and activity goals.

FXT has a unique and modular fitness structure that's built around your personal goals while using the extremely easy-to-follow FXT Point System for workouts. Once you've chosen your goal, you can follow our sample workouts while you learn how to develop your own programs for lifelong fitness. Whether they're short-term goals like rapid fat loss or sculpting your physique, or the long-term adoption of a healthy fitness lifestyle, these goals blend seamlessly from one program to the next without needing to employ an expensive personal trainer, purchase a gym membership or wait until "the time is right" for you to start getting fitter, healthier and happier with your appearance.

As your fitness changes and you progress through the program, you can target new goals such as speed, strength, muscle gain, definition/tone and even endurance for your first marathon or triathlon! Just follow the simple guidelines for adding or subtracting points to your weekly workouts and you have the roadmap to get you to your new destination.

Whether your goal is to drop a little extra weight, shave minutes off a marathon time or build core strength for a more powerful tennis serve, *Functional Cross Training* is the workout partner that will push you to your full potential. In addition to revolutionary day-by-day workouts, this illustrated guide delivers over 100 unique exercises, complete with step-by-step photos, that will enable you to transform your body and perform like you never thought possible. The only thing that's between you and achieving your fitness goals is taking the first step and getting started!

The Journey

Brett: My fitness journey started out way before I ever had the pleasure of meeting Jason, really back to when I was a little fat kid. When I look back at photos now, I realize I was probably just "chubby," but my self-esteem and body image were always pretty poor and I had an unhealthy level of resentment for the fact that many of my friends were fitter or more athletic than I was. I wanted to be better, faster and fitter, but I never had the desire, motivation or know-how to get started.

After college, I grew my hair and picked up a guitar and didn't exercise or play any organized sports until I met Jason in late 1999. During those 15 or so years, I'd gained well over 50 pounds and picked up smoking cigarettes, nearly two packs a day. Little did I know how much my life would change shortly after this hotshot programmer kid named Warner showed up at my office.

Jason: Brett and I became friends in the late '90s when we were working at an Internet start-up company. We became fast friends despite me being in my early 20s and Brett being nearly 30. We did things you'd expect brothers to do: played all sorts of sports, competed against each other in softball, football and basketball, and worked out together. It was some of the most fun I've ever had. From the beginning, we were both interested in fitness, though neither of us had a clue what we were doing. We thought we did, but hindsight lends perspective.

We had no clue, and the prevailing conventional wisdom didn't help, either. We ate and worked out just as the experts told us to, but we didn't seem to be getting anywhere.

We tried to learn. We did the very typical thing of grabbing all the fitness magazines we could find, reading them, tearing out pages and comparing notes. We quickly realized that fitness magazines were NOT in the business of educating people. In the same magazine you'd find several conflicting pieces of information—workouts that talked about doing the exact opposite of a workout only a few pages earlier and an eating style that was a huge no-no a few months ago. Even after our "research" we were left in the dark.

Brett: We were confused about what program to choose, so we tried everything

we could. With Jason's help, in the span of a year I'd dropped nearly 65 pounds of fat, met the woman of my dreams, quit smoking, and started down the path to fitness and a much healthier, happier life. Everything was going perfectly until life stepped in and Jason moved 2500 miles away. Gone was my source of knowledge and motivation, as well as my exercise buddy. It seemed like I was destined to head back to plopping my butt on the couch after work. It would've been so easy to put back on all the weight I'd lost, but now I was a totally different person and was proud of the changes I'd made, and I wasn't willing to give up.

Shortly after Jason moved away, I channeled the competitiveness we'd share each day on the basketball court or at the gym into a new addiction—triathlon and marathon running.

Jason: When I arrived in Phoenix, the new company I was working for offered us a free gym membership so I took full advantage of it. Moving to a new state with no family or friends and my wife working long hours during her medical school residency, the gym was practically my home. If I wasn't in the weight room, I was out on the basketball court. All of the high-intensity training was really starting to pay off and I found myself in the best shape of my life, right up to when I injured my Achilles tendon and was forced to change my routine and learn about rehab. I cover this a lot more in *Weights on the BOSU Balance Trainer*, but the bottom line was that I learned more about training during the period when I was rehabbing my Achilles than ever before. During this time I started developing very specific routines and drills for sports performance and made the choice to someday become a personal trainer.

Brett: It took about seven years for Jason to convince me to move out to Arizona, and during the time apart we'd developed completely different training regimens. Mine was all about speed, endurance and bodyweight exercises and Jason's included many more Olympic-style lifts, plyometric movements and strength-building exercises. While we were originally on opposite ends of the training spectrum, we sort of met each other in the middle to create hybrid routines that would work for a 150-pound triathlete and a 225-pound weightlifter. We didn't know it at the time, but it was the start of FXT.

Jason: Both of us are information sponges. Being reunited only reinvigorated our mutual love of all things sport and fitness related. We continued researching and experimenting with everything under the sun, trying to find what worked and what didn't. We spent time figuring out endurance training and nutrition, then we moved to strength and power training. We meticulously catalogued the things we did, making sure to note what worked and what didn't.

Both Brett and I became certified personal trainers right around the time we began to work on *7 Weeks to 50 Pull-Ups*. We took everything we'd learned about improving our physiques and weight loss and created the programs that would become *7 Weeks to Getting Ripped*. From there, I guess we went a little overboard.

Brett: Over the next two years, we developed programs and wrote books, everything from *Ultimate Jump Rope Workouts* to *7 Weeks to 10 Pounds of Muscle*. We authored programs for tackling obstacle courses,

triathlons, road races, medicine balls and BOSU Balance Trainers, and even worked with coauthors on nutritional programs for athletes, vegans and those following the Paleo diet.

Functional Cross Training, or FXT, is the culmination of all the programs—or at least all the "good" ones—we've developed over the last decade in one place. FXT is the result of years of learning the whats, the whys and, most importantly, the hows of fitness for the average individual looking to get fitter, faster and stronger. FXT is for everyone, no matter his or her goal. It's about teaching people and giving them the tools to actually understand what's going on with their bodies and how to craft a training and nutrition program for your specific goals. In short, FXT is about you and getting you to your goal, whatever that is.

Millions of visitors to our websites, countless e-mails and personal messages from you—the fans of our books, mobile apps and online programs—inspired us to continually develop and tweak FXT in order to deliver something truly new and unique to fitness that will help make it easier for you to get fit. This book and program is dedicated to each and every one of you out there who's looking to make a change and embrace a fitter, healthier and happier lifestyle. Thank you for your continued support, and we sincerely appreciate the feedback we've received over the years in order to build the most comprehensive yet simple training plan ever. We truly hope you enjoy it and develop a lifelong relationship with fitness!

About the Book

The *Functional Cross Training* program is designed to make selecting a program and sticking with it as easy as possible. Pick your goal-based program, choose the level that meets your age, weight or fitness level, and track your weekly workout points. It's that easy!

In **Part I**, we give you an overview of both functional and cross training, then show you how and why we mashed them up into an incredibly effective series of programs to build your strongest, fittest, fastest and healthiest body ever. We'll help you decode your goals and get you to focus on setting the right goal, as well as pair you up with the right fitness program to help you reach (or exceed) it as rapidly as possible. You'll find plenty of information in our FAQ section to help you get started or overcome some nagging doubts that are holding you back from getting fit, and then finally give you some motivation to get you on your way.

In **Part 2** you'll come face to face with the program that's custom-matched to you, addressing your goal, your level and your duration to reach your new level of fitness. We'll cover:

Fitness: How to build a fitness-based lifestyle

Speed: How to become explosively fast

Endurance: How to go farther, longer

Muscle: How to develop a sculpted physique with lean muscle

Strength: How to build the power to lift more weight

We'll also explain the easy-to-use point system for workouts and start you out with sample workouts to get you off and running (or lifting, squatting or even actually running). Based on your goals and adjusted for your current level of fitness, each program is simple to follow. It's even easier to create your own, with potentially millions of different workouts that grow and progress along with your fitness level to continually challenge and strengthen your entire body.

Of course, the workouts would be nothing without the exercises, and in **Part 3** we provide over 100 of them, with multiple variations to keep your body working through various planes of motion. They include bodyweight and weighted movements, dozens of core-sculpting exercises, plyometrics and so much more. Each exercise group is based on functional movements to develop rock-solid muscle in your upper body, core and lower body. This section also features warm-ups, stretches and cardiovascular drills to get you ready for the workouts, keep you loose, develop endurance, raise your metabolism and, of course, recover after each completed regimen.

Nutrition will also play a huge part in your lifestyle and physique transformation, so you'll get the lowdown on everything you need to know about fueling for performance—what to eat and when to eat it to maximize your training and get in the best shape of your life in **Part 4**.

If weight loss is one of your goals, turn to the **Appendix**. Here you'll get the lowdown on how to figure out how many calories you need on a daily basis. We also provide additional full-body exercises as well as a quick 10-minute travel workout that you can perform anywhere so you never have a reason to miss out on your workouts!

We've created and tested these programs over the last several years, and the goal of combining them all into *Functional Cross Training* is to make fitness accessible for everyone regardless of age, gender, weight and current level of physical ability. We hope you approach this book as a reference to create workouts of all types for years to come and, most importantly, we sincerely hope you have fun getting fit. After all, if you can't enjoy the journey, can you ever truly enjoy the destination?

What Is FXT?

Simply put, FXT, or functional cross training, is a multi-plane, multi-discipline and multi-muscle workout regimen designed to develop speed, strength, flexibility, athletic ability and full-body fitness. FXT was created to help athletes of all ages, sizes and athletic ability realize and meet their true fitness goals by blending real-world "functional" movements and cutting-edge full-body "cross-training" workout regimens into one dynamic program.

In order to understand the genesis of functional cross training, it helps to review the terms "functional" and "cross training" to get a clearer picture of how and why training with the FXT program can help you develop a higher level of performance and gain a deeper knowledge of the exercises and routines you can use for lifelong fitness.

Functional Movements & Functional Training

Functional movements are simple, real-world actions that we might take for granted...until we can't do them anymore: picking up a box, walking up stairs, navigating a shopping mall full of people. Functional movements are also things we don't necessarily do every day, such as swimming, running, hiking, carrying your children in the amusement park, dragging your luggage through the airport and stowing it in the overhead compartment. Functional movements can also take place in sports: chasing after a pop-up in baseball, spiking a volleyball, bounce-passing the basketball to a teammate or getting past a defender for a lay-up. Any motion that requires one muscle group to stabilize while another muscle group performs an action (flexion, extension, rotation, etc.) is a "functional movement." Most often, that stabilizing group is the core musculature—the abdominal, spinal and trunk muscles.

In order to train to perform functional movements, you need to perform full-body functional movements. While that's no huge revelation, so many of us spend an overwhelming amount of time trying to get in shape by focusing on very specific exercises designed to work a limited muscle group when we'd reap much more benefit from using our

Around 2006, Jason injured himself pretty badly when he tore his Achilles tendon. The next several years were filled with frustration and pain trying to get it back in shape. There was a period of time, right after his first child started to run around the house, that Jason realized how important simple things were. His Achilles wasn't healing properly and he began to wonder if he'd ever chase his son around the park, kick a ball with him, or even play a game of basketball as he grew. Forget rugby, marathons or 500-pound squats—Jason wanted to enjoy playing outside with his son! In order to rehabilitate his body, Jason had to essentially "start small" by focusing on small, everyday tasks and movements before he could participate in sports again; he needed to put the function first, and then focus on performance.

entire body to perform exercises designed to mimic real-world movements.

Functional training is essentially utilizing exercises that incorporate multi-joint, multi-muscle, full-body movement. The type of movement employed can differ from basic to complex but, make no mistake, this training style doesn't take place flat on a bench or require performing multiple reps targeting one specific muscle with one specific motion. Through different types of exercises, from walking to running or sprinting to calisthenics, functional training utilizes your own body weight as resistance through a wide range of movements to develop a fit, well-balanced athlete. All exercise that furthers the goal of pain-free movement and core stabilization can be considered functional training.

What does that mean? Getting stronger, becoming more agile, flexible, faster and fitter, and developing endurance are all examples of the positive byproducts of functional training. While you're working to improve your performance at particular kinesthetic functions, your musculoskeletal system is adapting, growing and changing to make your entire body more functionally fit.

What Is Cross Training?

Think of the most specific athletic movement possible. Is it shotputting, where the single goal is to throw something as far as possible? Is it running, where the goal is to pick up one foot and place it in front of the other? Is it doing the deadlift, where the goal is to pick up the most weight from the floor you can? All of these movements appear to use one particular discipline to perform each singular goal. Should those athletes train by only focusing on the distinct muscles used by each of those athletic movements?

One of the biggest mistakes athletes make is to take a myopic view of their training, isolating their body's overall function in terms of a specific goal. Running is a classic example of this. For years people training for a marathon would simply run, thinking that running for more miles and more time would get them in the best shape possible to run the marathon and complete their goal. This is no longer the case now that coaching, training and recovery/therapy methods have improved. Of course, someone hoping to finish a marathon needs to run a considerable amount, but to do it well they also need to work out with weights, train their core and not neglect their overall movement patterns. Specific training for a prolonged period of time, no matter the type, always leads to imbalances that will catch up to you at some point.

Athletes can improve specific sport-related performance by adopting exercises and training methods designed to promote full-body

Running is a perfect example of a linear activity, while everyday movements occur on multiple planes. How often have you heard a perfectly fit runner sidetracked by a pulled muscle from twisting to pick up a bag of groceries? When you train excessively in one specific plane, most other major muscle groups are neglected, as are the supporting muscles that "bridge" one group to another to allow fluid, balanced movements.

strength, flexibility and overall fitness. The term "cross training," used to refer to athletes in one sport adopting training methods from another sport during their off-season, is appropriately applied to athletes utilizing a multi-sport training regimen. They're essentially training their bodies to be as fit as possible in order to improve their overall athletic performance.

To think about it another way, the body is a very complex machine prone to failure. Optimal performance means making sure the entire machine is performing as it should. If someone trains only by running, the cardiovascular system is improving, lower body tendons are improving, and some lower body muscles are adapting to handle the stress of running. But your core is not improving and could actually degrade. What about muscular imbalances? Are they improving or degrading? Is this optimal training?

As another example at the other extreme, if a power lifter who only competes in the bench press event is training only for that specific event, what's happening to the rest of his body? Is his chest getting stronger than his back? Is he training his legs to support that added upper body weight? Is he doing any core training or performing cardiovascular training to improve his endurance? The answers to all these questions are most commonly "no," and his limited training methods that are extremely effective at crafting massive chest and arm muscles are also incredibly effective at developing an unbalanced physique and stressing or injuring other body parts, which are forced to overcompensate for the disproportionate growth in other muscle groups.

Of course, we're not suggesting that a runner and a power lifter should be training in even remotely similar fashion, though we are saying that both should be using a very balanced training approach geared toward their specific goal. To do otherwise is shortsighted and, frankly, dangerous.

It may sound counterintuitive but should make perfect sense: Cross training supports very specific fitness and athletic goals by strengthening the entire body in a balanced, safe and effective manner. By training the entire body to maximize performance and movement, each of the specific muscle groups needed for precise skill are improved. You may have heard the aphorism "a rising tide lifts all boats," and that holds true for your body. The fitter your entire body is, the better you can become at every athletic movement. All athletes, no matter how specific their goals, need to add multi-planar training to become fitter, faster and more flexible and perform better.

Why FXT?

FXT is about training smart for lifelong activity while being a simple, effective and adaptable program that you can use anywhere, anytime. FXT is about supporting your goal in an easy-to-follow, easy-to-implement, easy-to-continue fashion. FXT is also lifestyle training, perfect for families looking to get into shape together as well as athletes looking to improve in their specific sport. FXT is individual, modular and all-encompassing. FXT is for everyone. FXT is for you.

FXT works on the widest of fitness spectrums, from someone looking to move in a pain-free fashion to another looking to become a professional athlete. *Functional Cross Training* will furnish you with the information to actually understand why you'll be doing something. This book will offer the templates on how to achieve your goal. It will also provide you with the ability to adapt everything to you as an individual. With hundreds of different exercises and multiple different programs created for optimal performance at different athletic pursuits, FXT was created for athletes of all ages, sizes, and existing fitness levels to set, train toward, and meet their goals. Our pledge to you is that we'll do this in an approachable way that everyone can understand and follow.

The first step in the process is understanding and focusing on your real fitness goals. This is probably the hardest yet most important aspect of the entire process—athletes commonly skip this part, assuming that they already understand the goal they're working toward. In the section "What Are Your Real Goals?" (page 49), we break down some common vague targets and help you ask yourself the important questions about what you want to get out of your training, and then point you toward the program(s) that will suit you. Even if you think you know your goal, please take the time and read through the goal-setting section.

Once you've chosen and committed to your goal, we'll equip you with the background to understand why we advocate certain approaches, training styles and timing. Each of the programs for muscle, strength, speed, endurance, fitness and weight loss have their own very specific training method to get you on track to crush your goals as quickly as possible. With FXT you'll use total-body movements to develop total-body fitness that will benefit every aspect of your life, from basic, everyday actions to sport-specific conditioning.

FIT:FOOD—Fueling the Athlete

Nutrition is vital to developing a strong, lean, athletic body and performing at high levels in any sport, whether individual or team-based. Starting on page 169, there are two different nutritional programs, one for the specific needs of athletes building muscle and strength following the FXT:MX1 and FXT:ST1 programs, respectively, and also one distinct program for the athletes following the FXT:FIT, FXT:SXP and FXT:EXP programs. Both nutritional regimens are aligned with the goals of each of the programs. Turn to the Appendix on page 181 to determine your BMI and BMR and how many calories you need for your size, weight and sex, and then make those "calories" work for you by making excellent macro- and micronutrient choices to fuel your body for athletic performance. (On page 169, you'll see why we added the quotation marks to calories.)

Getting to Know Your Body

Some of us (ahem, Brett) are the type of folks who like to learn by doing. Whether it's jumping from the roof of the garage or sticking a fork into an electrical outlet, you don't need to know why something is a good or bad idea, you just want to go for it and figure it out along the way. We can't vouch that this is a good method, but it's the way some of us tend to do things, come what may. Others among us (like Jason) love figuring out why things work the way the do. This next section is for cerebral types like Jason who like to understand all of the proper terms and calculations you may need during your journey. For the rest of us, you can use the rest of this chapter as reference material.

Body Movements

Before we get into the programs, let's cover some anatomical terms and body positions that will be used in the exercise descriptions in Part 3. No one's going to test you on the correct use of any of the terms, but it's really helpful to have a general idea of what they mean. This is barely more in-depth than the "foot bone's connected to the ankle bone..." song—it's just a few points of reference.

Range of Motion (ROM): This is the entire spectrum of movement allowed by one's anatomy and physiology; limits are based on joint, muscle, ligament and cartilage positioning, size, shape and condition— essentially the mechanical limit you could possibly move if you were in top condition. Training to strengthen your musculature and develop more flexibility will allow your joints to function with as wide a ROM as possible. While range of motion technically covers hyperflexion, hyperextension, etc., those conditions are not considered optimal. Therefore, when a trainer uses the phrase "complete the movement with as full a range of motion as possible," this doesn't include putting your joints in a hyper-anything position.

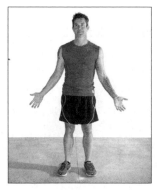

Anatomical Position & Planes of Movement: The anatomical position is essentially the "default position" for your body as nearly all joints are in neutral position with the exception of your elbows (which are rotated forward to bring your palms onto the frontal plane)—feet face forward and are about shoulder-width apart, spine is erect, arms are extended at the sides of your trunk with palms facing forward. The three different anatomical planes of movement are median, frontal and horizontal, and all are described by starting with the anatomical position. The median plane splits your body laterally into right and left halves with a vertical line through your belly button (the medial line). The frontal plane splits your body into front (anterior) and back (posterior) sections when viewed from the side, bisecting your torso vertically in a line that runs through your ears, shoulders, hips and ankles. The horizontal plane splits your body into upper (superior) and lower (inferior) halves at your belly button. Most motions in life are a combination of these planes.

Athletic Position: Similar to anatomical position, this is often described as the "ready position" for many sports. We'll refer to this in nearly every exercise where you're on your feet. In a standing position, your feet face forward and are approximately shoulder-width apart and slightly rotated outward (laterally) about 10–15 degrees for greater balance. Knees, hips and elbows are slightly bent (commonly referred to as "softening your joints"), and arms are rotated slightly forward at the shoulders. This position should have you ready for quick

TIP: Don't confuse athletic position with the "ready position" of some sports. For example, a shortstop will have a far deeper knee bend and hip drop to allow for a more explosive lateral or vertical movement when the ball is hit.

action or reaction in any direction, primarily a median or horizontal plane.

Flexion & Extension: Often confused, these are relatively easy to remember once you get the general mental picture. Flexion is accomplished by bending a hinge (elbow, knee) joint, while straightening a hinge is extension. Forcing one of these joints past straight is considered hyperextension, and commonly responsible for serious injuries. Note the word "general" above—you can also extend and flex at the hip and shoulder (ball and socket) joints without bending; raising your arm or leg forward and upward is flexion, while returning it to anatomical position is extension. The neck, wrists, fingers and toes all get in on the flexion and extension action, but you get the general idea and you're not getting quizzed.

Rotation: You'll be using this one quite a bit, primarily when twisting the trunk. Simply put, this rotation is bringing the side of the body bisected by the frontal plane toward the medial plane while traveling along the transverse plane. Sorry, couldn't resist. In other words, you're rotating your trunk so one of your shoulders is aligned with your belly button. Easy, right?

Abduction & Adduction: Abduction of the hip or shoulder joint occurs when the leg or arm is lifted outward (laterally) from anatomical position; your shoulder has a much wider range of motion than your hip—shoulder abduction encompasses the entire lateral movement upward of your arm from your side to directly over your head. Adduction is the motion of bringing the arm or leg back to anatomical position. We use a little mnemonic to differentiate between the two: "Abby opens."

The Muscles behind the Movements

The exercises in this book are designed to work all major muscle groups and most ancillary muscles in your body. Now, we're not going to go into great detail of all of the 640 muscles you happen to possess, so we'll break the body down into two main sections: "movers" and "core."

Movers are any muscle whose prime movement is to push, pull or rotate any part of your body aside from your core. The core is the foundation that allows the movers to do their thing and handles twisting and crunching. The stronger your core is, the more effective, efficient and enduring all your mover muscles will be. Building your core strength is the key to total-body fitness and absolutely imperative when developing a fit, ripped physique along with functional fitness.

Throughout the book, we'll focus on exercises that use at least one from each group. Most will use both, and many will use nearly all of your muscles. We've covered this before, but let's repeat it just to be sure: In order to become functionally fit, you'll need to train multiple muscle groups on multiple planes. Got it?

MAIN MOVERS: UPPER BODY

Pectoralis Major: This pair of thick, fan-shaped muscles makes up the bulk of the muscle mass in the chest. The "pecs" are responsible for rotating, flexing and bringing in both arms for actions such as throwing a ball, lifting a child, or performing jumping jacks or push-ups.

Triceps Brachii: The large muscle located on the back of the upper arm, the triceps brachii (commonly referred to as "triceps") is responsible for straightening the arm. The triceps makes up over 50 percent of the upper arm's muscular mass.

Deltoid: This heart-shaped muscle group is made up of three different fibers (front, middle and rear). While each fiber type has a specific function, the "delts" as a whole are responsible for raising and stabilizing the arms during rotation.

Biceps Brachii: One of the assisting muscles during a pull-up, the biceps brachii (commonly referred to as "biceps") is responsible for forearm rotation and elbow flexion. It's located on the front of the upper arm. *Note:* Chin-ups are more effective at targeting the biceps than pull-ups due to the supinated grip.

Trapezius: Another prime mover, the trapezius (commonly referred to as "traps") is a large, superficial muscle located between the base of the skull and the mid-back, and laterally between both shoulders. Its primary function is to move the scapulae (shoulder blades) and support the arm.

Latissimus Dorsi: The latissimus dorsi (meaning "broadest muscle in the back") is responsible for moving the arm toward the center of the body (adduction), internally rotating the arm at the shoulder toward the center of the body (medial rotation), and moving the arm straight back behind the body (posterior shoulder extension). It also plays a synergistic role in extending and bending the lumbar spine to either side (lateral flexion). This pair of muscles is commonly referred to as the "lats."

Forearm Flexors/Extensors: The structure between the elbow and wrist contains a number of muscles, including the flexors and extensors of the digits, brachioradialis (which flexes the elbow), pronators (which turn the palm of the hand downward) and supinator (which turns the palm of the hand upward). These muscles allow you to grip the bar during a pull-up.

MAIN MOVERS: LOWER BODY

Gluteus Maximus & Minimus: These muscles make up the majority of the buttocks and are responsible for maintaining an erect posture, raising from a squat position and performing most leg motions, such as adduction and rotation. *Note:* The glutes are a crossover core/lower-body muscle group and often neglected. Without strong glutes, your body would lack the power to get up out of a chair and walk! See the section on the core for more on the importance of developing your backside.

Quadriceps: The quadriceps ("quads") is a large muscle group made up of four muscles on the front of the thigh. It's the strongest, leanest muscle mass on the body, responsible for straightening the knee joint and crucial in walking, running, squatting and jumping.

Hamstrings: The hamstrings, located on the back of the thigh, are made up of four muscles responsible for knee bending and hip straightening. The hamstrings work as antagonists to the quadriceps to enable walking, running and jumping, as well as maintaining stability in the hip and knee.

Calves: The triceps surae, or "calves," is made up of the gastrocnemius and soleus muscles. These muscles attach to the Achilles tendon and are responsible for ankle rotation, flexion and stabilization, and are crucial for walking, running and jumping.

CORE

The term "core" refers to the area of the torso composed of the rectus abdominis (the "six-pack" portion of the abdominals), obliques, transversus abdominis, and erector spinae, but there's much more to it than that! Your glutes, as well as hip flexors and extensors, play a huge role in core strength. When most people think of a strong core, they immediately picture six-pack abs, when real core strength comes from all the other muscles that make those eye-popping abs possible. Full-body functional movements originate from this area of the body, and a strong, flexible core provides stabilization during every activity your body performs on a daily basis, from performing a pull-up to maintaining proper posture when walking, standing or sitting. A strong core is essential to proper fitness—your body's strength needs a solid base to work from.

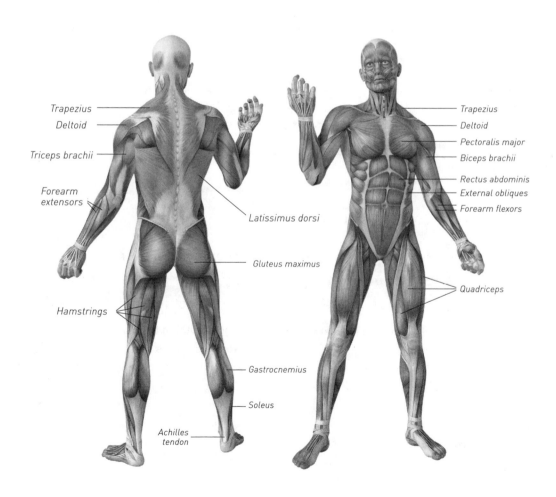

Trapezius

Deltoid

Triceps brachii

Forearm extensors

Latissimus dorsi

Gluteus maximus

Hamstrings

Gastrocnemius

Soleus

Achilles tendon

Trapezius

Deltoid

Pectoralis major

Biceps brachii

Rectus abdominis

External obliques

Forearm flexors

Quadriceps

Frequently Asked Questions

Q. Can I do this? Is it doable?

A. Absolutely. We have both proudly smashed our personal goals, overcome plenty of mistakes and missteps, and continued to tweak the program to get positive results and surpass what we expected to accomplish. You can too.

Q. What's the single best tip you can give to someone about to start this program?

A. Create realistic goals ahead of time and stick with the program until you meet them. Whether it's doing 20 sit-ups or 200, losing 5 pounds or 50, or building the strength in your core to help eliminate lower back pain and straighten out your posture, commitment, focus and follow-through are the most effective methods to reach your goals. See "What Are Your Real Goals?" on page 49. Remember, no one expects you to be a pro at every movement. Some exercises may come naturally while others feel completely foreign. All you can do is keep working on perfecting the form and get stronger along the way. Don't give up and sit out an exercise if you can't do it—make the investment in yourself and learn the proper form for each move. You'll only reap the benefits.

Q. How can I find time for a workout? I walk to work, uphill both ways, in the snow, without boots...

A. Yes, we all have real life to keep us busy and it can be difficult to sneak a workout in on a regular basis. Actually, YOU are the one making it difficult. Yeah, we're pointing our fingers squarely at you, and defy you to prove us wrong. Without any question, you have 15–20 minutes to spare three times a week to improve your physique and feel better about yourself and you know it's true. Wake up a few minutes earlier, go to bed a few minutes later, cut down on your TV watching or web surfing, and you'll be surprised how easy it is to make sure you don't miss a quick workout. If you need some help remembering, set a calendar reminder or use a mobile app like the one we developed as a companion to this book (shameless plug). The bottom line is: You can find the time quite easily if you want to, and you want to, right?

Tip: Work out for half of your lunch break three days a week. If you get an hour, use 30 minutes to warm up, work out, cool down and clean up and you'll still have plenty of time to eat the (healthy) lunch that you packed. It only takes a little planning to make this work, so make it happen!

Q. I already work out at the gym. Would I get anything out of this?

A. Absolutely! The exercises and workouts here would make anyone a fitter person, not to mention a better athlete. Who can't use a stronger core, more balanced and stable musculature and better body awareness? Both the muscle-building program and the bodyweight exercises can absolutely be done in any gym, whether it be at home, in a hotel, a CrossFit box or any health club. Obviously, the weighted workouts need the appropriate dumbbells or barbells that you'll find at a gym, and most have one or more pull-up bars, exercise mats and sit-up benches too. With a little creativity, ANY gym or space is a great workout area!

Q. I have an injury. Can I still work out?

A. See your doctor. Boring answer, but the truth. The workouts are rigorous and the addition of weights and high intensity could make some very common injuries worse if you're not careful. Above all else, be safe and see your doctor first before performing any demanding physical activity.

Q. I have a bad knee/shoulder/elbow/hip. Can I still follow the program?

A. Have you seen your doctor? No, seriously—go see your doctor before you start any fitness or nutrition program. Since you'll be lifting your body weight or additional weights, it'll be important for you to have as much full range of motion, a stable base and balance in your musculature as possible. A ripped ACL will greatly affect your ability to perform heavy squats, and a rotator cuff injury will surely hinder presses, rows...you get the idea. While we provide some alternate exercises, injuries are surely going to hamper your ability to perform certain movements. Be smart, lift within your ability and let injuries heal before pushing too hard. You're going to have this body for the rest of your life—there's plenty of time to recover and pack on muscle when you're ready.

Note: If you skip squats and deadlifts, you're limiting your ability to pack on muscle. It's just the facts: Multi-joint exercises are a big part of the mass-building protocol.

Q. Should I be sore after every workout?

A. Soreness may be normal if you're a beginner, have recently changed up your routine or are trying a new activity. The initial soreness should lessen over time; it's not normal to be sore after every workout. If you continue to be sore, you may need to take more days off between workouts. Soreness after running depends on your age, conditioning, the intensity of the workout, terrain, form and countless other factors. The good news: It usually gets better as you adapt to a program. The bad news: As you're progressively pushing yourself to reach new goals, you'll continue to develop soreness after a workout. Post-exercise stretching,

recovery and rest will help you alleviate some soreness. The best tip is to get eight hours of restful sleep. We cover some ways to maximize your downtime on page 38.

Q. How should I breathe for each movement?

A. For many of the exercise descriptions, we'll cover when to breathe in and out, but overall it's a good idea to breathe out when you're exerting the most force (pushing, pulling, etc.) and breathe in on the recovery. Breathing properly is a big part of being able to perform some of the main exercises we'll be covering in this book, so make sure to focus on breathing rhythmically and never holding your breath during sets.

Q. How quickly should I do the movements?

A. Some exercises will have specific speeds during certain workouts, but as a rule of thumb you should try to stick to a "medium" speed. Listen to your body; you'll know what's too fast or too slow with a little bit of experience. If you're just learning the movements, take them as slowly as you need to maintain proper form. Some exercises or drills like sprints will require a specific percentage of maximal effort and speed. When it's necessary, we'll call it out in the instructions.

Q. Will all the workouts be an effective way to lose weight?

A. Any exercise above what you're currently doing aids in the goal of losing weight and getting into shape. The programs in this book utilize the fat-burning benefits of circuit training and high-intensity interval training (HIIT) to help you lose weight and get into fantastic shape while developing your total body. When paired with balanced nutrition, you'll be firing up your metabolism in as little as 20 minutes a day to burn excess fat and shred your physique.

Q. What days work best for following this program?

A. Again, this is up to you, but we've found over the years that the success rate goes up exponentially if you pick three days during the week to perform a structured program like the ones featured in this book. In order to get the optimal rest of 48 hours between working the same muscle group again, we recommend scheduling your workouts on Monday, Wednesday and Friday.

Q. What's the best time of day to do the workouts?

A. That's totally up to you, your goals and your daily schedule. We actually recommend performing the weight-loss program in the morning before eating to maximize the fat-burning effect of training while your body is burning about 60 percent fat as fuel, which happens during sleep and when you first wake before eating. In the muscle-building program, we showcase some different exercise and nutrition timing to maximize benefits. Most of the workouts in this book are designed to be done almost anywhere, so pick a time that works for you. You could do sets of exercises while you get ready in the morning or after you get the kids to bed.

Q. What's the secret to success with any of these programs?

A. Commit the time and effort to doing the program right. Often it really helps to have a partner (that's how we created the programs!) who'll keep you on track to complete the

workouts. Mark workout days on your calendar, set an alert on your computer or smartphone for the short amount of time the program takes. You can do what we did back in 2008 when we started these programs—block your calendar from noon to 1 p.m. each day to make sure you get uninterrupted exercise time.

Q. What's this "rest" thing you keep talking about? Have you seen my schedule?

A. If you don't rest, you won't recover. If you don't recover, you lose most of the benefit from your workout. I use the term "most" because you still burned some extra calories during the exercise and raised your heart rate to obtain some cardiovascular conditioning benefit...but if you don't rest, well, you'll miss out on the benefits of building lean muscle.

Q. Is it possible to just work off my love handles?

A. Yes, but the answer might be different than you think. The secret to losing your love handles is to train your entire body using bodyweight exercises. Want ripped abs? Train your arms, back, shoulders and legs...and your abs will reap the benefits.

Q. How many days a week should I work on my core?

A. There's a long-standing myth that your core can be worked every day. Let's take a moment and address that: When you place any muscle under repeated stress from lifting weights (time under tension) or repeated movement, microtears begin to form. These extremely small tears in the muscle fibers are actually a positive benefit of working out; when they heal, your muscles grow bigger and stronger. In order for muscles to properly recover, heal and grow, you should wait 48 hours before working out that same muscle group again. Now, we ask you, what's your core made up of? Your rectus abdominis, erector spinae, obliques, hip flexors, quads, glutes and hamstrings are all muscles and need to rest, recover and grow.

Q. Can't I just do crunches to rip my abs?

A. You can do crunches all day long and still not have a ripped core. Period. Unless you work your entire body to get lean, you just won't be able to show off your six pack.

Q. I was always told to stretch first, but lately I've read that you shouldn't stretch your muscles when you're cold. What's the deal?

A. Research and studies over the last few years have reinforced the reasoning that you should warm up before you exercise and then stretch after you've completed your workout. Read more about warming up and stretching on page 166.

Q. I've seen other muscle-building programs. How does this differ?

A. These programs provide a linear approach to training, offering people programs that they can use their entire life. These programs also combine the approaches that make other programs successful and reject the fluff that causes frustration. Simply put, this is as cutting edge as it gets for hypertrophy programming.

Q. I'm confused whether to use bodyweight exercises or weighted movements to develop my physique and increase muscle size. Can you help me decide?

A. Reading through "What Are Your Real Goals?" on page 49 should help you decide where to start, but here's a little overview: If you want to build the biggest muscles possible, loading up a bar and doing reps of weighted workouts in the muscle-building program (page 116) is the way to go. But, remember, you can build huge arms, chest and legs and still be unable to perform well at the complex motions necessary for many sports. Using a blended approach of weights and bodyweight exercises, you'll build your entire body, and the end result will be a stronger, faster and fitter version of you. You'll also be amazed at how much bigger muscles look when you're ripped.

Q. Can I just build bigger biceps using the muscle-building program?

A. No, these are all full-body programs, not designed to target any particular muscle group. You'll get bigger arm, leg and chest muscles, and whatever overall gains you make will be spread over your entire physique.

Q. How long is it going to take me to build muscle?

A. It depends on your goals, your drive, your metabolism...and a whole other host of factors (age, sex, testosterone level, muscular imbalances, training ability), not to mention the most important factor—having a life.

Q. Can I do a full-body workout every day?

A. No, your body needs time to rest and recover. When you do strength-training exercises such as pull-ups, you create tiny, harmless tears in the muscle. These tiny tears heal during rest days. As a result, the muscle becomes stronger and more defined. If you don't allow the muscles to heal, you risk overuse injuries that could potentially derail your ability to exercise at all. Constant repetitions of any motion without proper rest will eventually result in overuse injuries. Repeat this sentence: "Rest is equally as important as the workout for strengthening and shredding your body." Now, make sure you follow your own advice.

Q. Will full-body strength training make women bulk up?

A. The bodyweight exercises in this book were selected specifically for men and women to develop lean, shredded bodies, and the muscle-building program is geared toward developing strong, solid muscle. Typically, women don't have the kind of hormones necessary to build huge, bulky muscles and thus need to follow a very comprehensive nutrition and supplementation program to do so. Full-body strength training benefits both men and women by creating leaner tissue and losing any excess fat (by increasing metabolic efficiency), slowing muscle loss (especially in older adults) and decreasing risk for injury.

Q. Can I combine other workouts with these programs?

A. If you're an athlete who needs to train sports-specific skills, then the workouts in this book should be used to supplement that training. If you're hoping to quickly get stronger or more ripped by doing extra workouts on "rest days," then you're in danger of overtraining and not letting your muscles rest, recover and grow. For best results, follow the program that you've chosen—rest included—from start to finish to maximize the results. Don't develop "Workout ADD" and jump from one program to the next.

While any exercise with good form is a positive for your body, willy-nilly exercise-picking will not necessarily provide the targetable results you're looking for.

Q. Should I lose weight before I start running?

A. Why not let running help you lose weight? The FXT:PX1 (page 71) is an easy way to get into the swing of a routine and will help you walk, jog and run at your own pace to help lose weight and prepare you for advancing to any of the other programs down the road. The best part? It's all relative. You can use any program for as long as you need while you build up your strength and athletic ability and drop weight before progressing.

Q. Can I run every day?

A. Eventually, yes—but you need to build up your endurance and strength first. Experienced runners who lace up every day will vary their workouts between tempo runs, intervals, hill work, easy runs and longer distances to keep their body and mind fresh. Too many intense workouts back to back can lead to burnout, overuse injuries and overtraining. Too much of a good thing is still too much, and trying to do excessive amounts too soon is a sure way to knock you off track with injury or boredom. See "Overtraining" on page 35.

Q. I heard that running is horrible for my knees/back/spleen/nostrils/etc.

A. Life is hard on your body, running isn't. Actually, the health benefits of losing weight, adding muscle and increasing your cardiovascular system's efficiency far outweigh the wear and tear on your body from being active. Running is an activity, and all activities increase your potential for injury. That's just the nature of the game.

Q. It's too hot/cold/rainy/hilly where I live. Can I do some of the cardio or drills on a treadmill?

A. Sure! Running outside can be a little more exciting than being stuck on a "dreadmill," but we know plenty of runners who log thousands of miles on their treadmills and achieve great results at races. The benefits of getting a run in without worrying about weather-specific clothing can be a big plus when you're strapped for time. One tip: Always change the elevation of your treadmill deck to at least 1 or 1.5 degrees to reduce the flat-footed impact on the belt that can lead to shin splints.

Q. I don't have enough time to run or exercise!

A. Yes, you do. That 5 minutes you waited in line at Starbucks, 15 minutes on Facebook before lunchtime and 60 minutes spent spacing out while pretending to be working would be a perfect time to sneak in a couple miles or even a few sets of bodyweight moves. Get creative with finding spots where you can sneak a run or workout in, and then clean up, change and return to your daily activities. Don't have a shower? Bring some sport wipes (like baby wipes, without the baby smell) and a little deodorant. They work pretty well!

Q. I missed a couple scheduled workouts or runs. Do I have to start over?

A. We all miss workouts. The most important thing is to get back on your program as soon as you can. Work, family, illness, travel, holidays, injuries and plenty of other forces are collaborating against your planned exercise. It happens! If you miss a week, start from where you were. If you miss more than that, keep moving back your workout the same amount of time you missed. At about two weeks you begin to lose some of the base fitness and running acumen that you've built up.

Q. I was able to follow my program very well early on but am now having trouble doing the required reps. What's going on?

A. Initially, your body goes through a number of changes when you start a new program. Your body will soon begin to adapt to the workouts; you'll notice a plateau once you become used to doing any exercise. These programs have been carefully designed to avoid this plateau effect by changing the duration, intensity and workout routine over seven weeks. Follow your program as best you can. In the unlikely event you do hit a plateau, continue to follow the plan and eventually there'll be enough change to get you over the hump. Remember, don't overdo it and be sure to take the necessary rest between workouts. Every two months we want you to reflect on your success and progress and re-evaluate your goals and program choice. Mixing it up and changing programs after eight weeks is a proactive way to avoid hitting plateaus.

Before You Begin

Guess what? We're going to tell you to get off your ass and go to the doctor before you start this (or any) fitness program. How does right now work for you? Chances are, you're a 20-minute visit away from a clean bill of health. Even if the doc does find anything alarming, you're much better off catching it early than having it sneak up on you later.

Brett's wife Kristen absolutely forbade him from training for Ironman Arizona in 2009 until after he received his doctor's sign-off, and he's glad he did. Hundreds of hours running, biking and swimming would've been a foolish undertaking had he not had his ticker checked out first. Suck it up, make a call and go see your doc.

As for Jason, remember when he said he tore his Achilles? After it "healed," he wanted to train and play rugby but had some nagging questions: Could his Achilles handle not only the training, but the stress of cutting on the field? Was he setting himself up for another tear? Was his Achilles weaker than before the injury? A quick visit to the doc cleared all that up. Had Jason NOT done that, he would've been worrying about every little ache and pain every time he stepped into the training room or onto the field. Visiting the doc and clearing his doubt allowed Jason to perform optimally.

Want one more reason to go see a doctor before you start? She'll give you some encouragement in your new pursuit of fitness (or at least she should) and when you come back for your next visit she'll be able to say, "Wow, you look great!" and maybe even pat herself on the back for getting you to follow doctor's orders!

If we didn't yet make it perfectly clear: Always obtain clearance from a doctor that you're healthy enough to begin this or any other strenuous exercise regimen. Perform each exercise within your ability and always use proper form (page 40). Most of all, don't be stupid and try to do too much, too fast—that's a recipe for a pulled muscle, injury or a bout of DOMS (see page 33) that will knock you off track from completing the next workout.

Listen to Your Body

You should be able to tell when you're ready to begin fitness programs like these by tuning in to your body. Take it easy and be smart about determining what's normal soreness from a workout and what's a nagging injury that you're aggravating. If you think it's the latter, take a few extra days off and see if the soreness passes. If it doesn't, you should see a medical professional.

You should expect to experience mild soreness and fatigue, especially when you're just getting started. The feeling of your muscles being "pumped" after a workout or a hard run and the fatigue of an exhausting workout are normal, as is the flush of warmth when finishing a challenging set of intervals. These are positive feelings. On the other hand, any sharp pain, muscle spasm or numbness is a warning sign that you need to stop and not push yourself any harder. Some muscle groups may fatigue more quickly because they're under-trained or have been unused for a while. Every muscle in your body will be taking on a tremendous amount of new work and can easily fatigue. Your joints and feet are taking a lot more of a workload than they're used to and will surely become sore. If you feel uncomfortable and can't run or exercise anymore, take a break, walk or catch your breath and grab a sip of water. If you're really beat, light-headed or dizzy, stop immediately, rest and rehydrate. Get medical attention immediately if those symptoms persist or you feel any of these heart attack symptoms:

- Discomfort, pressure, heaviness or pain in the chest, arm or below the breastbone

- Discomfort radiating to the back, jaw, throat or arm
- Fullness, indigestion or a choking feeling (may feel like heartburn)
- Sweating, nausea, vomiting or dizziness
- Extreme weakness, anxiety or shortness of breath
- Rapid or irregular heartbeats

MUSCLE SORENESS

Once you begin any of the programs in the book, you'll be performing it at your own pace and within your personal level of fitness. If you're new to working out or returning to exercise after some time off, be sure to take your time and take it easy for the first two weeks to allow your muscles to adjust to the new workload and reduce post-workout soreness. Delayed onset muscle soreness, or DOMS, is the soreness you experience 24, 48 or more hours after pushing a workout too hard. This will hamper, limit or completely sabotage your program. You have plenty of time to get in the groove with these programs, so take your time and work your way into them!

You can keep DOMS at bay by using these two guidelines:

1. Don't overdo any muscle group, especially if it hasn't been targeted by a workout in a while. For example, take it easy on squats, deadlifts and lunges right off the bat or you'll have quad/glute/hamstrings that feel like concrete the next day.
2. Make sure to keep active the day after a workout and keep your muscles loose. No, this isn't a workout—just take a walk or do jumping jacks to warm up and perform some stretches like the ones

you'll find on page 166, accompanied by activating the sore muscles by moving them through as full a range of motion as possible.

This may come as a shock, but no one's perfect at every exercise when they get started—usually far from it! Even after some practice, you still won't be a pro at every movement. Some exercises may come naturally while others feel completely foreign, and almost all exercises take a long time to fully master. Multi-joint, multi-muscle movements like squats are already complicated and difficult to master with just your body weight; when you perform them with weights or at high intensity they're a much more demanding, yet rewarding, exercise. It's extremely important to keep working on perfecting the form and get stronger along the way. Don't give up and sit out an exercise if you can't do it—make the investment in yourself and learn the proper form for each move. You'll only reap the benefits.

If you feel extremely fatigued or have an uncomfortable level of pain and soreness, take two to three days off from the workout. Some muscle fatigue and soreness is to be expected and you can continue to exercise carefully when you're a little tired or sore. Any sharp pain, pinches or throbbing aches in your joints is not to be ignored. If the discomfort or pain persists, seek the advice of a medical professional. If you feel any sensation in a joint or muscle that makes you say "uh-oh," then stop immediately, rest and assess whether or not it's a serious injury that needs medical attention.

Due to the nature of a full-body workout routine, you'll be lifting, pushing and pressing your entire body weight along with the occasional additional pounds in your hands. It's very important that you focus on proper form and utilize the proper muscles to complete each exercise. This means no cheating by arching your back on push-ups or allowing your knees to bow in during squats—you're only cheating yourself. Every proper-form rep just gets you closer to your goals!

If you have a pre-existing condition like joint instability or a muscular imbalance, make sure you recognize any physical limitations, take your time and work your way up slowly while focusing on training with good form. It's far more important to be careful with nagging injuries than it is to worry about completing all the exercises in any specified amount of time. Performing the exercises with proper form will help you to build strength, flexibility and balance, as well as improve your sports performance—but not if you ignore the warning signs and hurt yourself. If pain or soreness persists, please see a medical professional.

When performing any exercise routine that requires you to lift, pull or press your body weight, don't take any chances with unsafe equipment. In addition, make sure you're properly trained to use any equipment before you start a workout. Always be aware of your surroundings and make sure you have plenty of room to execute moves safely without hitting or tripping over other objects.

ANTI-INFLAMMATORIES

It's been said that "ibuprofen is an athlete's best friend," but it's extremely easy to become too reliant on "vitamin I," causing health issues and even slowing your body's natural ability to heal. Inflammation is a normal part of the healing process when your cells essentially attack an "injured" area by increasing blood flow to speed up recovery. The swelling and pain associated with inflammation aids in healing, but also exacerbates the discomfort.

During training, performing the exercises creates small micro-tears in your muscles. When running, it happens with every single step you take. The harder or longer you train, the more stress is put on your muscles and the more micro-tears you'll have. While a muscle tear sounds like a bad thing, these micro-tears are actually good, as they help your muscles to strengthen and grow as they heal. The inflammatory response that's signaled by this muscle damage causes your body to deliver more blood, oxygen and nutrients to immediately begin the healing process. An anti-inflammatory (non-steroidal anti-inflammatory drug, or NSAID) can actually impede some of this rapid healing. Furthermore, an over-the-counter anti-inflammatory can mask some of the symptoms of more acute muscle strain or pain that could be signaling you to stop working out because there's some damage. You can't listen to your body if you're trying to get it to shut up and stop nagging you!

NSAIDs do have a positive role in reducing pain for short periods of time if you experience something like a low-grade sprain or somewhat sharp joint pain. With any severe pain, see a doctor immediately. Stop training and rest for one to three days while following the prescribed dose on the NSAID's bottle. After three days, reduce the dosage and let your body heal itself. Relying on an anti-inflammatory long-term can prevent you from healing and also potentially damage your kidneys if taken in prolonged heavy doses. If you have any questions, call your doctor.

MIND-BODY CONNECTION

A fancy phrase used to describe awareness of your own body, muscles, movements and reactions is "kinesthetic awareness." As we age, this musculoskeletal and mental connection often declines, though hope is not lost! Kinesthetic awareness is trainable, and by harnessing the power of FXT, you can—and will—reconnect with your body.

This leads to our next fancy word: "proprioception." Proprioception describes how your body reacts and responds to external forces to keep your joints in the correct position. When performing proper-form bodyweight movements, nearly all of your muscles are forced to contract to keep your joints in the proper position.

Don't think this is a big deal? Quick test: Stand on one foot with your other foot off the ground and close your eyes. Now just try to stand there for as long as you can. You see, in normal circumstances, we need vision to help us balance—this is natural. Closing your eyes makes you need to be aware of your muscles, and you need to actually focus on the balancing, with only your muscles reacting to the way your body is positioned. For most people this is incredibly difficult. After some practice you'll be able to control even the small muscles in your body. This added awareness and control will help in all manners of your daily life.

This goes for all movements, from running to weightlifting to walking. Be keenly aware of your body: feel the movements and stresses, understand the muscle firing, feel the foot landing. The mind-body connection helps you stop going through the motions of an activity to feeling it and understanding what's happening, catching potential injury issues early and ultimately performing better.

Overtraining

The easiest way to spot overtraining is when you've trained successfully for a while and suddenly your results start to drop, along with your energy and desire to keep on training. Guess what: This is your body telling you to stop! Too much of a good thing is still too much, and overtraining can quickly unravel all the gains you've gotten out of your efforts over the past few months.

Put simply, overtraining is training too hard and not allowing physical and mental recovery between workouts. The symptoms manifest as physical, behavioral and emotional stress that limits the athlete's ability to make progress and can begin to diminish any strength and fitness gains made. While it's normally problematic in weight training, it's common in runners and athletes of all types as well. Too much of a good thing is a bad thing—you can absolutely run and train too much to your own detriment!

Overtraining may be accompanied by one or more concomitant symptoms:

- Persistent muscle soreness and fatigue
- Elevated resting heart rate and reduced heart rate variability
- Increased incidence of injuries
- Irritability
- Depression
- Irregular sleep patterns
- Mental breakdown

Note: We've indulged in this type of behavior. Not only have we both overtrained from time to time while creating new routines for multiple books, we even went so far as to support too much of one particular exercise in our first collaboration, *7 Weeks to 50 Pull-Ups*. Now, in our defense, that book is a "challenge" versus a comprehensive training program, but the end result is still the same—too many pull-ups and not enough of...well, anything else. Just remember, that book is centered around a challenge to complete more pull-ups than ever before and not a full-body regimen. (Phew, that feels good to get off our chests.)

This goes to show that overtraining is nothing to be trifled with, and the best way to combat it is by lowering your training volume or upping your rest and recovery time. (Check out "Rest & Recovery" on page 38.) Here's our formula for preventing overtraining and maximizing recovery—the 6 Rs:

RUN/TRAIN

REFUEL

RECOVER

REST

REPEAT

RE-EVALUATE

Run/Train three to five days a week based on your physical ability and previous conditioning. Beginners should take every other day off or put in a relatively light effort while more advanced athletes can mix in one or two "off days" per week.

Refuel (immediately, if not sooner). Follow the directions (starting on page 174) for nutrition before and after specific workouts as some will differ slightly. For example, after a hard run lasting more than 90 minutes, drink a beverage that contains a 4:1 carb-to-protein ratio. The carbs help to replace the glycogen you burned off for energy while also shuttling the protein to your muscles to speed recovery. For muscle-gain programs, you'll be taking in protein and carbs before, during and after workouts in a completely different ratio.

Recover with post-workout stretching, foam rolling, an ice bath (if you're brave), a trip to a steam room, a dip in a whirlpool or a warm tub with some dissolved Epsom salts. You can also slip on compression socks, or even get a full-body deep-tissue massage. We can only personally vouch for the post-workout stretching, foam rolling and deep-tissue massage as being extremely beneficial to a faster recovery, but we'll never pass up a chance to sit in the hot tub. The jury is still out on compression socks, so try them for yourself if you're interested.

Rest for at least eight hours a night, and be sure to use your off days as off days—not time to sneak in additional workouts! Get tips that pro athletes use for developing good rest habits on page 38.

Repeat as necessary. You can't stick with a program unless you keep at it until it becomes second nature. By maximizing your rest and recovery, you also greatly increase the odds that you'll be ready, willing and eager to tackle your next workout. However, you need to continually look for signs of overtraining or developing a nagging injury. It's your responsibility to make sure your body can handle the workload and continue.

Re-evaluate your program every two months. Are you progressing with more reps, more intensity or heavier weights? Are you reaching your goals and is your performance improving? How do you look and feel? Don't be afraid to modify your program based on your individual successes or failures—the only goal of FXT is for you to develop the fitness you want. Re-evaluate your specific program and make changes as needed to your workout schedule or intensity; you might even switch which program you're using. One note: Modifying your program does not mean skipping a body part (unless you're recovering from an injury) or avoiding an exercise because it's not fun. These are still workout programs designed for total-body functional fitness.

RHABDOMYOLYSIS

While DOMS from pushing your workout intensity too hard, too fast is uncomfortable and often results in three to five days of soreness that will limit nearly all physical activity, it's not life threatening. Rhabdomyolysis, on the other hand, is extremely severe and can result in long-term muscle damage, kidney failure and death. Yes, you read that right: An extremely intense workout can actually kill you if you push your muscles past their limit for expansion and contraction (usually rapidly) and inflict damage to the muscle fibers, causing muscle cells to disintegrate, releasing the waste product from those cells into your bloodstream. Immediately, your liver will start trying to clean your blood and, when it becomes overwhelmed, it can cause renal failure.

Throw the phrase and underlying theory "No Pain, No Gain" out the window—too much pain can destroy the exact muscles you're trying to grow, and much worse. All of the programs in this book have been designed to work within the normal parameters of average athletes; you control the intensity, number of reps and heaviness of weights used in your own program. While there's no specific threshold for all individuals where muscles are taxed beyond their ability to continue to function and break down, it's generally limited to several dozen repeated exercises that continue well past muscle exhaustion. While we encourage you to push through your barriers for speed, endurance, muscle growth, strength, and athletic performance, we're not encouraging you to do it with reckless abandon.

Follow the guidelines for each workout as best as you can, depending on your own existing athletic ability. It's much better to perform a slow, controlled workout than it is to rush through just to beat a specific time. Slow, gradual progress is far more beneficial than a short-term gain that results in an injury.

Rest & Recovery

When do your muscles grow? In or outside the gym? It's an easy question to answer, but harder to put into practice. Your muscles grow when you're not in the gym. Technically they mostly repair themselves when you're sleeping, so take naps, get eight hours of sleep a night and make sure you get adequate rest between workouts.

The programs will call for four workout days and three rest days. USE ALL THE REST DAYS! Don't be tempted to "just work out a little" on those days. Give your body time to heal. We're going to be throwing quite a bit at you pretty quickly. Take advantage of all the time off allotted. Each program features a different exercise and rest schedule, and you need to follow the proper rest and recovery just as diligently as you follow the workout regimen! Not only will you be at risk of overtraining or a repetitive stress injury, you won't be giving your muscles time to heal and grow properly.

Here are some tips to keep in mind:

- Get at least eight hours of sleep every night. This includes weekends too. Your circadian rhythms are easily knocked off-balance by late-night partying (or book writing).

- Minimize any exercise or activity within one hour of bed. By the time you hop into the sack, your heart rate should be at a resting level.

- Turn off your electronic devices. Living rooms are for TVs, bedrooms are (mostly) for sleep. Leave your mobile device, laptop or tablet in the other room; lit-up screens have been shown to disrupt early sleep patterns and keep you from falling asleep quickly. Falling asleep with the TV on generally means you'll stay up far later than you intended and only nod off when the infomercials start airing, right?

- Turn off your brain too. Your bedroom should be a peaceful, relaxing sanctuary where you sleep and escape from all your stresses. Worrying does not promote a restful state, and you most likely won't fix your issues while you're in bed. Maximize your mattress-time effectively by getting quality sleep.

- Set the scene for rest. Keep your room dark with heavy curtains to block as much light as possible and use a fan or noise machine to provide a soothing sound to lull you to sleep.

- Fuel your body to build muscle during sleepytime. Protein provides the critical amino acids that serve as building blocks for the formation of new muscle. Casein and whey are the two non-soy protein powders you'll find at nearly any grocery or health-food store. While whey is metabolized quickly and should be taken immediately after a workout, casein protein is metabolized slowly and perfect for keeping your body anabolic while you're asleep.

Learning & Using Proper Form

How important is using proper form when performing an exercise? Let's just say it's not important at all—if you want to derail your workout by pulling a muscle, tearing a ligament, breaking a bone or any number of bad outcomes. Not only is there the vastly increased potential of you really hurting yourself, you'll also be getting less benefit from the workout.

Let's think about this logically: Why would you bother to move around heavy weights or perform numerous bodyweight exercises while risking injury and get virtually no benefit after all that time, sweat and hard work? If you're working out with improper form, that's exactly what you're setting yourself up for.

What Is "Proper Form"?

Every single movement has what can be described as "optimal" form, when the body's musculoskeletal system is aligned in such a way to most efficiently support itself, move a specified range of motion or transport weight from one position to another. In the simplest of terms, proper form can be seen as a scale with "optimal form" at one end of a continuum and "dangerously poor form" at the other. Proper form is as close to optimal as possible, and without hesitation we can say that no one uses optimal form all the time for every exercise. Now, that's not to say that optimal isn't the end goal of exhaustive practice and training, and the closer you get to this pinnacle the more you'll reap the benefits of proprioception, strength, flexibility, speed, lean muscle definition, endurance and every other fitness goal.

In reality, we all need to learn the basics of proper form for each exercise and build up to executing each with as few flaws as possible as we progress to become better athletes. You should strive for perfection while understanding that good/proper form is the baseline you should employ to execute each movement.

Of course, there's not one universal measure of proper form for every movement (that'd be too easy, right?). Each exercise has its own specific body position, range of motion, balance and alignment points that dictate proper form for that exercise only. Note that there are plenty of similar exercises (some even with the same name!) that require significantly different elements of form.

Below are some very good examples of the different variations of the weighted squat. Though they're all squats, they require very specific—and different—movement and form, target muscles, range of motion, weights, etc.

As you can see, the name "squat" refers to the vertical movement and stabilization and lifting of weights (body weight, barbell, dumbbell, etc.) but each movement has

EXERCISE	MUSCLES TARGETED	WEIGHTS	IMPORTANT FORM DIFFERENCE
Back Squat (page 148)	Quads, Hips, Glutes, Core	1.5x your body weight	Bar is on traps, which puts more stress on lower back. Sit back as you would sit into a chair. Keep torso upright; don't lean forward; drive through your hips and glutes.
Front Squat (page 149)	Quads, Core	.75x–1x your body weight	Hold bar high and tight on your front delts near collar bone. Be sure to keep torso very upright and try to go straight up and down.
Bulgarian Split Squat (page 151)	Quads, Glutes	.5x–.75x your body weight	Rear foot is either up on a bench or behind you. Front foot is firmly grounded via the heel. Lower until you feel a stretch in your back-leg hip flexor. Pause and push up through your front heel.
Goblet Squat (page 148)	Quads, Hips, Core	.5x your body weight	While holding a weight at chest level in front of you, sit back and lower down. Drive up through hips and glutes. Puts less stress on the lower back and more on the core.

different body positions to target different muscles through modified plans of motion. One singular squat definition does not do any of the variations justice. Naturally, proper form for each of these moves is unique and needs to be learned and repeatedly practiced.

The bottom line is you'll need to take many movements, if not all of them, step by step with the descriptions (see Turkish Get-Up on page 135 for a great example of this) and employ a mirror or a workout partner to check your body position to make sure you're getting all the benefit of each exercise while also limiting your exposure to injury from improper and dangerous movements.

What Does Proper Form Look Like to You?

No matter how well we're trained, each of us has some certain nuances to our form that may be suboptimal. Whether they're bad habits or muscular imbalances, they can be robbing you of potential strength, muscle and fitness gains, reinforcing the imbalances in your musculature or even setting you up for injury. The best option would be to work with a partner (preferably a certified trainer) who understands proper form and can guide you through exercises and give you tips to keep you on the proper planes and let you know when your form is failing. If that's not an option, set up a video camera or your smartphone to film 2–3 reps with a weight you can lift comfortably more than 5 times—too light and you may be masking some poor form by muscling up an easy weight; too heavy and you may hurt yourself.

Once you've worked through your form, it helps to remember what the proper motion feels like by repeated practice and developing muscle memory. Here are some tips that help remind us to continually focus on perfecting our form.

Jason: Where do you put your hands on the bar when you bench press? Outside the lines? Middle finger on the line? Pinky? How about several inches inside the lines? Which one is "right"? Instead of thinking about hand placement, try thinking this: "I want a long, healthy, pain-free life. How can I make sure I maximize my gains while minimizing pains?" I used to put my hands outside the lines as I felt it really focused the tension in my chest. As the weight got heavier (remember, muscle grows faster than ligaments and tendons), little muscle tweaks and dull joint pains started. I quickly realized it wasn't sustainable. Over the past few years I've taken a completely new approach to my form. As an example, I now take a much narrower grip with the flat-bar bench press: my hands are shoulder width (pinkies on outsides of shoulders), elbows tucked (NO FLAILING ELBOWS!). I also pause at the top with straight arms. Think of it as in between a narrow-grip and wide-grip bench press. Though it may sacrifice both weight on the bar and muscle isolation, I can lift more pain free and for the long term. I've found this is much more sustainable and, frankly, enjoyable. I'm in this for the long haul and don't need to blow out an elbow doing something that clearly isn't working.

Brett: Even after all my training with Jason to learn all the movements for *7 Weeks to 10 Pounds of Muscle* and working through every exercise over a multi-month test period, I was surprised to get feedback from a fellow trainer during a workout. Frank Sole (a collaborator on *7 Weeks to a Triathlon*) walked over during my final set of squat cleans and asked me what the heck I was doing with my head. My leg, back and arm position was great (according to him) but he couldn't figure out why I was looking straight down at the floor instead of keeping my neck relaxed and eyes level. Apparently, I was focusing so much on looking at the bar to make sure I was doing the lift right, I was putting my neck in a stressed position...and for the past few weeks I thought my pillow was the cause of my stiff necks each morning!

Some Dangers of Bad Form

We've already warned you that you're risking injury to muscles, joints or tendons by lifting heavy weights or performing multiple repetitions using poor form, but there are some other factors that may make you think twice about perfecting your body position and movement for each exercise.

Bad form results in bad results. You won't be targeting the proper muscles that the exercise or program is designated for if your form is off. For example, the angle of your torso when lifting a weight makes all the difference between, say, an incline chest press, which develops your pectoral muscles, and a front shoulder press, which works your deltoids.

Bad form results in injury. No surprise here. When you put your body in an awkward position (more on that below), you're more prone to pulling, tearing or breaking things that have no business being incorporated into that movement. For example, performing squats with your knees bowed inward more often than not results in knee strain, pain and even meniscus damage.

Bad form results in you looking like an idiot. Let's just be honest—anyone who falls off a ball is going to illicit a snicker from even their closest friends and workout partners—not to mention the rest of the gym faithful! (Of course, that's as long as you don't get hurt; no one should ever laugh about that.) All kidding aside, it's acceptable to struggle with a new and difficult exercise until you get it right, especially when it's a challenging unbalanced movement. It's another thing altogether when you watch someone struggling through an exercise with too heavy a weight or with really bad form. Unfortunately, unless someone corrects them or they do a little online or written research or "gym reconnaissance," they'll stick to the same improper form and wind up a candidate for one of the top two bullet points above.

TIP: Gym reconnaissance is used by many, but sometimes it's a recipe for disaster. Just because that gal over there with the amazing abs does her medicine ball wood chop that way doesn't mean her form is perfect. Do some research online or pick up a book and make sure you know what you're doing before you adopt her style. On the flip side, if you see someone absolutely struggling and making the exercise look more like a battle than a movement, you should probably not adopt his style. Even difficult exercises should be controlled, normally fluid motions.

What's Your Motivation?

Let's face it—some days we all feel like we need a good reason just to get out of bed in the morning. We have a great gig writing books and training some awesome folks, but there are plenty of times when we'd like to smash the alarm and bury our heads under the covers. Workouts are the same way for most people—if they can think of any reason to skip it, they probably will.

We'll admit to missing our share of workouts, but it never seems to be worth it: when we skip one, we just ending up paying for it later with a subpar performance at a race or during a game, or even feeling miserable because we feel like we've let ourselves down. Usually the penalty is worse and lasts longer than the workout would've anyway. Brett's wife can always tell when he's cranky and has even thrown him out of the house to go for a run and cheer up—and it actually works!

Ninety-nine percent of the time, we feel like superheroes after a good workout. Our endorphins are all cranked and we feel absolutely bulletproof. If we could bottle that experience we'd be millionaires... but more importantly, if we just remind ourselves how great we'll feel when we're done with the training, it makes it that much easier to get psyched up for it. The remaining 1 percent of the time we either forgot our gym shoes or something. It happens to all of us.

Often misattributed to Beethoven, Ignacy Paderewski mused, "If I miss one day of practice, I notice it. If I miss two days, the critics notice it. If I miss three days, the audience notices it." Fitness is similar yet not exactly the same as a world-renowned musician skipping out on hours of playing scales. We all miss workouts, that's a given; the goal is to find your motivation and make it to far more than you miss.

The bottom line with motivation is that you'll never get through any life change without it. You need to be motivated to change jobs, try a new restaurant, even brush your teeth. Some motivation is easier (and smellier) than others, but every modification to your course of action requires you have the incentive to give it a shot and the follow-through to stick with it.

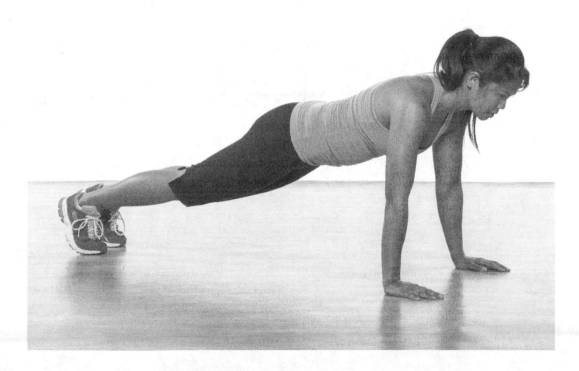

Here we introduce what we like to refer to as the "ass-ivation" scale, progressive levels of motivation, from getting active through developing athletic performance:

Get off your ass-ivation: This is the most common motivation with individuals as they become more sedentary. It will usually involve an epiphany after finishing off a bag of chips on the couch or just not fitting into your favorite jeans anymore. No matter what Mick Jagger sang back in 1964, time is not on our side, and every day, month or year you spend inactive, you're gaining weight, losing athletic ability, stamina and cardiovascular fitness and letting your body go to pot.

Lose my ass-ivation: This is weight loss and toning, usually for a life event like a wedding, beach vacation, class reunion or newfound single status that forces you to look somewhat presentable to others. "Boot camps" are really popular with this group because people are usually looking for immediate results.

Kick some ass-ivation: This involves athletic improvement or sport-specific training for an upcoming season or events. Speed, core strength, endurance and flexibility are a common focus for most sports that involve getting from point A to point B as rapidly as possible, especially athletic endeavors where you repeat that over and over (e.g., soccer, football, baseball, paintball, etc.).

Now, these top-three "ass-ivation" goals aren't mutually exclusive. You can lose weight, get healthy, improve your athletic ability and develop a fantastic physique all at the same time. Heck, that's what FXT is based upon! Using the "What Are Your Real Goals" section (page 49), you can begin your preparation and kick your plan into gear.

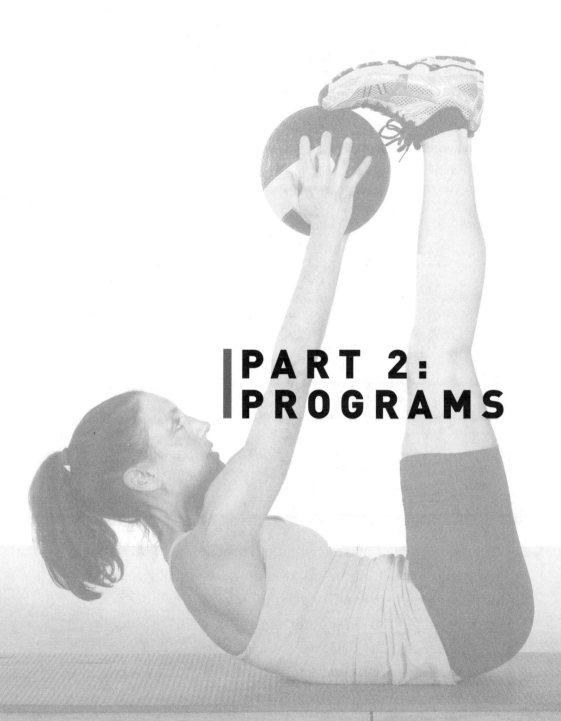

PART 2: PROGRAMS

Getting Started

"If you don't know where you're going, you might end up someplace else." —Yoga Berra

Here's where the revolutionary program for developing a toned, muscular body while maximizing athletic ability comes into play: We've created simple-to-follow, amazingly effective, goal-driven fitness plans for every individual regardless of age, weight or current physical ability. In other words: FOR YOU. Here's where the rubber meets the road, and we define each of the goals and your weekly points.

What Are Your REAL Goals?

The single most-important thing to getting results you'll be happy with is actually understanding what you want to achieve. What is your actual goal? Nothing else matters. Do you want to look like a cover model? Be honest, say so and understand that your program and diet will differ from your neighbor/partner/ friend who wants to run a marathon. Do you want to deadlift 500 pounds? Do you want to lose body fat? Do you want something you and your family can do together?

Want to know something awesome about goals? They're liberating. Having a goal frees you from worrying that you aren't doing something right, or you should be doing something else or more or slightly different. Having the goal allows you to be prepared to understand what's pertinent to your goal and what's not. Having the goal will give you a framework in which to view the rest of this book and see what applies to your goal and what doesn't.

Conversely, NOT having a goal is chaotic. We're going to provide too much information too quickly over a broad range of topics. All this information does not apply to every goal. Being firmly rooted in your goal allows you to filter information.

Set a goal. Now. Stop reading and walk around. Think about it critically. What do you want to achieve? What are you looking to do next? When you picture yourself a year from now, what is Future You doing that makes you the happiest? What do You look like?

This is where the fun starts. Have your goal? Great. Now what's your REAL goal? Think of it this way. If someone tells us they want to

have a six-pack, we know immediately that their real goal is to lose body fat. Everyone has a six-pack, but not everyone is lean enough for it to be seen! Conversely, if someone tells us they want to look like a cover model/ action-movie star, we know the goal is more complex. They'll likely need to gain muscle and later lose body fat to show off the new muscle. Similarly, someone who says their goal is to run a marathon has a real goal of building endurance, leg strength, likely losing weight and preventing injury.

Real goals are the basis for achieving your goals. It's equal parts understanding, honesty and fortitude. You'll need to understand what it takes in both nutrition and workouts. (We'll provide this in later chapters.) You'll also need to be honest in all phases of the game. Be honest with yourself about your REAL goal (you're only cheating yourself otherwise), your ability to adhere to the diet, your ability to adhere to the workouts required and your ability to stick to timelines. Last, but without doubt the most important, thing is fortitude to see it through.

We can guarantee very few things, but one of them is that at some point you'll want to quit or cheat or think you're making progress and stop. You need mental fortitude to push past this and keep going. Those moments are the most critical to your long-term success. In the beginning, those moments are likely few and far between as you're excited about something new and can picture it. The challenge comes later when you hit your first wall or stall. Don't stop. Never stop. These are the moments when dreams are tested and goals are shattered. Keep going, push through, dig deeper, find the inspiration and motivation. When you look back a year or two from that moment, you'll either be happier and healthier or you'll be in the same rut you are now. Progress is always moving forward.

DECODING YOUR REAL GOALS

Now that we've talked about goals and REAL goals, it's time to decode your REAL goal into a plan. We'll provide the tools and framework for the plan, though only you can know your individual REAL goal to put the plan into action.

Here are quick sample templates to decode your REAL goal. It's strongly encouraged you do this exercise with pen and paper.

SAMPLE 1

You say: "I'm a 45-year-old guy with a beer gut who wants to lose 25 pounds and run a 5K in six months."

You mean:

- 45-year-old male (required for assessing BMR, THR, BMI)

- Out of shape (good for determining program level)

- 25+ pounds overweight (specific, measurable goal)

- Run a 5K (specific, measurable goal)

- 6 months (specific, measurable time frame)

How you'll get there:

Step 1: Assessments

- Visit your doctor and make sure you're physically ready to participate in a fitness routine (see page 31).

- Measure your BMI, BMR, THR, etc. (see page 182).

- Test your physical ability, range of motion, cardiovascular conditioning, strength, etc. (see page 58).

Step 2: The Program

Depending on the results of your test above, you'll either follow FXT:PX1 on page 71 or jump right into FXT:FIT (page 77) for 8 weeks and follow that up with FXT:SXP (Speed & Performance, page 89) or possibly FXT:EXP (Endurance & Long-Distance Performance, page 103). Six months provides ample time for three 8-week programs!

Step 3: Create your future.

- Learn how each of the FXT programs can be used to build a comprehensive, easy-to-follow, lifelong regimen to develop and maintain optimal fitness.

- Understand off-season, building, conditioning and strengthening, and how they all fit together.

- Re-evaluate your progress and goals; change programs, weights, duration or intensity.

- Have an active life. Seriously—functional fitness means very little if you're not using it by playing, hiking, biking, jogging, swimming or just being active.

SAMPLE 2

You say: "I'm a 35-year-old new mom. I want to get back to my pre-baby weight and tone up a bit in the process."

You mean:

- 35-year-old female (required for assessing BMR, THR, BMI)

- Baby weight from pregnancy

  Note: This goal lacks specificity. A rephrasing of this to be more achievable would be "I'm a 35-year-old new mom. I want to get back to my pre-baby weight of 135 pounds, but this time want to be more toned. I'd like to be the same weight (135 pounds) but 20–22% body fat."

How you'll get there:

Step 1: Assessments

- Visit your doctor and make sure you're physically ready to participate in a fitness routine (see page 31).

- Measure your BMI, BMR, THR, etc. (see page 182).

- Test your physical ability, range of motion, cardiovascular conditioning, strength, etc. (see page 58).

Step 2: The Program

Based on the results of your assessment fitness test, you may start with FXT:PX1 on page 71 or choose FXT:FIT, FXT:SXP or any of the other programs that suits your long-term goals.

Step 3: Create your future.

- Learn how each of the FXT programs can be used to build a comprehensive, easy-to-follow, lifelong regimen to develop and maintain optimal fitness.

- Determine baseline numbers (body fat to measure).

- Understand how to build muscle while losing body fat.

- Map and plan your future month by month for your time goals.

- Measure and track on a regular basis to make sure you're progressing.

- Re-evaluate your progress and goals; change programs, weights, duration or intensity.

- Have an active life with your family! Enjoy your newfound fitness by playing, hiking, biking, jogging, swimming or just being active, and motivating family members to do the same thing.

SAMPLE 3

You say: "I'm a 25-year-old skinny guy who wants to build muscle and look like a cover model."

You mean:

- 25-year-old male (required for assessing BMR, THR, BMI)

- Underweight, little muscle mass, low strength (good for determining program level)

Note: This goal lacks specificity. A rephrasing of this to be more achievable would be "I'm a 25-year-old skinny guy who wants to add 15 pounds of muscle and have 12% (or less) body fat by the time I am 27 years old."

This new goal means:

- 25-year-old male (required for assessing BMR, THR, BMI)

- Underweight, little muscle mass, low strength (good for determining program level)

- 15 pounds of muscle (specific, measurable goal)

- 12 % (or less) body fat (specific, measurable goal)

- 27th birthday (specific, measurable time frame)

How you'll get there:

Step 1: Assessments

- Visit your doctor and make sure you're physically ready to participate in a fitness routine (see page 31).

- Measure your BMI, BMR, THR, etc. (see page 182).

- Test your physical ability, range of motion, cardiovascular conditioning, strength, etc. (see page 58).

Step 2: The Program

Based on the results of the test above, you may be ready to jump right into the FXT:MX1 program (page 116) or spend a little time getting ready with FXT:PX1 on page 71.

Step 3: Create your future.

- Learn about muscle-building workouts and nutrition.

- Determine baseline numbers (body fat to measure, strength to track gym progress).

- Understand what causes muscles to grow while minimizing fat gain.

- Map and plan your future month by month for your time goals.

- Re-evaluate your progress and goals; change programs, weights, duration or intensity.

SAMPLE 4

You say: "I'm an 18-year-old college football freshman who wants to improve overall strength, lose weight to 10% body fat and improve my 40-yard dash time from 4.9 seconds to 4.7 seconds for summer training camp, which is six months away."

You mean:

- 18-year-old male (required for assessing BMR, THR, BMI)

- Athletic, lean and fast (good for determining program level)

Note: This goal lacks one vital piece of information: starting weight and body fat. It can be inferred from a 4.9-second 40-yard dash that you're a conditioned athlete, but you could conceivably be as high as 20% body fat.

This new goal means:

- 18-year-old male (required for assessing BMR, THR, BMI)

- Add strength (good to know strength focus vs. muscle size)

- 4.7-second 40-yard dash (specific, measurable goal)

- 10% body fat (specific, measurable goal)

- 6 months (specific, measurable time frame)

How you'll get there:

Step 1: Assessments

- Visit your doctor and make sure you're physically ready to participate in a fitness routine (see page 31).

- Measure your BMI, BMR, THR, etc. (see page 182).

- Test your physical ability, range of motion, cardiovascular conditioning, strength, etc. (see page 58).

Step 2: The Programs

Based on the "athletic, fast and lean" description above, you can make the jump right into FXT:FIT for eight weeks and follow that up with FXT:SXP Speed & Performance. From there, you can re-evaluate whether to repeat FXT:FIT or FXT:SXP with higher intensity to hit your goals. Six months is ample time for three 8-week programs.

Step 3: Create your future.

- Learn about strength and explosive conditioning as well as proper nutrition to fuel gains while losing fat.

- Determine baseline numbers (body fat to measure, strength to track gym progress).

- Understand what causes muscles to grow vs. strength to increase while minimizing fat gain.

- Map and plan your future month by month for your time goals.

- Measure and track on a regular basis to make sure you're progressing.

- Re-evaluate your progress and goals; change programs, weights, duration or intensity.

SAMPLE 5

You say: "I need to get in shape. I'm [insert age here] and [insert number of pounds here] overweight and I'm sick and tired of being sick and tired when it comes to my fitness. Help!"

You mean:

- "I have no idea how to get into shape."

- "I need help!"

- "HELP ME!"

What this goal lacks in specificity it makes up for in honesty. More often than not we've all felt lost and needed help and guidance from others to make a change in our lifestyle that will benefit us greatly over time. Often, it's extremely difficult to reach out for help and to make the sometimes-difficult decisions to get started. Once the barriers come down and egos are pushed aside, aspiring athletes are met with a ton of contradictory information on what's the "best" plan for them and they get lost in the mix and end up worse off than where they started. Well, that's not happening here. This new goal means:

- Show me a step-by-step exercise and nutrition routine so I can slowly transform my life. Period.

How you'll get there:

Step 1: Assessments

- Visit your doctor and make sure you're physically ready to participate in a fitness routine (see page 31).

- Accept the realization that there's no such thing as a quick-fix diet/pill/miracle cure that can transform your body composition, fitness level or life.

Step 2: The Program(s)

- Start with FXT:PX1 on page 71.

- Follow the nutritional guidelines on page 169 in conjunction with the program.

- Take your time and work through the program, progressing at your own level. You've started on a plan that will help you make the changes to adapt your lifestyle to fitness, or fitness to your lifestyle. It only takes a series of small changes over time to have a profound and lasting impact on your health and well-being.

Step 3: Create your future.

- Re-evaluate your long-term goals.

- Measure your BMI, BMR, THR, etc. (see page 182).

- Test your physical ability, range of motion, cardiovascular conditioning, strength, etc. (see page 58).

- Pick a program that suits your goals and get to work!

Goals are great. As we said earlier, they give you a framework to filter information and map your own programs to your individual needs. FXT is about providing a way for people, no matter their starting points, to locate pathways to achieve their goals.

Now it's your turn to say your goal out loud. Take some time and determine your REAL goal. Know it inside and out. Be honest with yourself. Feel your future, see yourself six months or a year from now and visualize that you've achieved or are on your way to achieving your goal. See your future self and assess if that's indeed your REAL goal. Do this as many times as you need until you know in your heart that your REAL goal is exactly what you want.

Picking Your Program

FXT is not just one workout program—it's actually several different goal-oriented programs under the umbrella of using functional cross training to become fitter, faster and stronger. We offer programs to develop speed, strength, endurance, general fitness, weight loss and muscle. Read through the overviews of each program to get a feel for which ones apply to your current fitness level and where you're looking to progress to, then match one or a series of successive programs to your specific goals to get yourself on track for the results you're seeking. As you saw in samples 1, 2 and 4 in "Decoding Your REAL Goals" ("Decoding Your REAL Goals" on page 50), each of the programs is designed to work together toward progressive strength, speed, endurance, fitness and muscle development.

Here's a cheatsheet that illustrates the overview of each program, how they all build on each other to create a progressive series, and what type of athlete can benefit most from each.

Program Cheatsheet

FXT:PX1 (page 71)	BEST FOR
General fitness, weight loss, introduction to performing bodyweight exercises with proper form and developing a fitness-based routine for an active, healthy lifestyle.	• All beginner or intermediate athletes looking to increase their fitness level, become more active, and lose weight and body fat while increasing lean muscle. • Athletes returning to training after time off or rehabbing an injury.

FXT:FIT (page 77)	BEST FOR
Prerequisite: FXT:PX1, or scoring highly on FXT:FIT test on page 60 Engineered for developing improved athletic ability, strength, flexibility, power and a lean, sculpted physique that's less prone to sports-related injury. Using bodyweight, plyometric, and weighted exercises, FXT:FIT is an extremely well-rounded program that can easily serve as the basis for all other training in this book or an excellent stand-alone program for athletes of all ages. Used with sports-specific training, this program incorporates full-body conditioning routines that can seamlessly enhance off-season, pre-season and mid-season training.	• Experienced athletes who are familiar with training techniques and are functionally fit, having completed FXT:PX1 and scored well on the FXT:FIT test on page 60. • All athletes looking to develop total-body strength and flexibility featuring a strong core and building a base in order to develop speed (FXT:SXP) and endurance (FXT:EXP). While not a required starting point to build muscle (FXT:MX1) or strength (FXT:ST1), this program provides an excellent basis for all types of training programs and exercise regimens.

FXT:SXP (page 89)	BEST FOR
Prerequisite: FXT:FIT Created to build explosive speed by using full-body training coupled with plyometric movements and drills, FXT:SXP uses functional cross training to develop speed in multiple planes, thereby making athletes stronger and more resistant to sports-related injuries.	• Short-distance runners and athletes in all sports requiring quick bursts of speed, changes of direction and sports-specific movements such as jumping, kicking, diving, sprinting, etc. • All athletes looking to develop progressive cardiovascular fitness, strength, speed and flexibility after completing FXT:FIT.

FXT:EXP (page 103)	BEST FOR
Prerequisite: FXT:FIT, FXT:SXP This high-intensity program has been created for athletes looking to develop prolonged strength and speed for elite levels of athletic ability—longer than that of their fellow competitors. Endurance refers to performance at an extremely high level for challenging events such as obstacle races (OCRs) and mud runs, trail marathons, triathlons and high-intensity team sports such as soccer, football or rugby.	• Experienced, extremely fit athletes competing in extremely challenging endurance events or looking to improve their fitness, strength and durability to compete at very high levels for a prolonged duration.

FXT:MX1 (page 116)	**BEST FOR**
Designed to build lean muscle mass as quickly as possible, this program is both an intro to using proper form in weighted exercises for beginners and an advanced program for experienced athletes since all weights are relative to the individual's strength and ability. Based on very specific lifting styles and a unique nutrition program designed to push muscle-building proteins into overdrive. Developed with all athletes in mind, FXT:MX1 is geared toward exposing athletes to many different lifting styles and workout types while teaching proper form for weighted Olympic lifts and other muscle-building exercises.	• All athletes looking to pack on muscle mass—particularly lean muscle.
FXT:ST1 (page 123)	**BEST FOR**
Prerequisite: FXT:MX1 As a follow-up to FXT:MX1, this program utilizes a very specific set of Olympic lifts using heavy weights in order to increase one's level of total-body strength.	• Experienced athletes who have mastered proper form on Olympic lifts while completing the FXT:MX1 program. • Individuals looking to increase their maximum-weight lifts, specifically their 1RM (one repetition maximum), while building a dense, solid physique.

How All the Programs Tie Together

Based on the goals you said out loud earlier (you did do that, right?), the chart on page 55 should quickly assist you in choosing the proper program. As you can see by the hierarchical structure of prerequisites, each program builds on a functional cross-training foundation to develop all facets of enhanced athletic performance, fitness, health and physique.

Beginning with the FXT:PX1, we provide two distinct paths to follow. One focuses on building a lean, ripped physique that maximizes power-to-weight ratio in order to improve athletic performance, cardiovascular endurance and speed. The second stresses packing on muscle mass quickly and developing the strength to push, pull and press heavier weights than ever before. The nutrition and fueling used during FXT:MX1 and FXT:ST1 (page 176) are geared to build more muscle mass and strength, and have a specific quantity and timing that's considerably different when compared to FXT:FIT.

Continuing the theme we started with the specific nutrition, the FXT:FIT, FXT:SXP and FXT:EXP programs have a great deal of overlap in terms of bodyweight and weighted exercises, drills and training methods. For instance, you'll see hill repeats or the 20/20 Drill (and others) in all three, but there are distinct differences in the ways these exercises and drills are used to develop very specific strengths and meet specific goals. FXT:MX1 and FXT:ST1 use nearly all of the same Olympic lifts, yet the speed and number of repetitions, amount of weights used and time under tension, and specific grips and body position will vary between the programs. Quite simply, when using FXT:MX1 to build muscle, you're targeting specific muscle groups in order to maximize time under tension, muscle stress, and growth. FXT:ST1 is about utilizing your entire body as a lever to lift as much weight as possible; this progressive resistance means the weight you're lifting should get heavier from workout to workout as you work toward increasing your maximum lifts.

Each of the FXT programs requires hyperfocus on form and completing the entire workout with high athletic intensity. To that end, we've added a "mantra" for each, courtesy of one of our athletic heroes, Dean Karnazes: "Struggling and suffering are the essence of a life worth living. If you're not pushing yourself beyond the comfort zone, if you're not demanding more from yourself—expanding and learning as you go—you're choosing a numb existence. You're denying yourself an extraordinary trip."

To keep track of your progress, we recommend that you make a few copies of the program log you're following, or download the mobile app for workouts on the go.

Baseline Testing

Once you've figured out your true goals, the next step is to get started...but only after you've had an appointment with your doctor for a checkup. Seriously, it's really that important that you get the all-clear before beginning any exercise regimen. It's much better to know—good or bad— than to find out during training or racing.

During Brett's first marathon, he raced with a coworker, Dan, who'd trained the same distances and speed as the rest of his group and was completely prepared. On race day, Dan inexplicably began to slow in the later miles due to shortness of breath, not the normal cramps or leg fatigue. A few weeks later, after still feeling drained daily, a routine exam led to the discovery that Dan had a hole in his heart that required multiple operations to fix. The doctor gave him some very chilling news: "You very easily could've died out there on the course." Not the news Brett wanted to hear as his running partner, but far less so something he or a course EMT would've liked to explain to Dan's wife and kids. Please see a doctor first, OK?

We've all got to start somewhere, right? This is the time and place to get on track with a FXT program that's perfect for you. Once you have your goals, it's time to take either the FXT:FIT or FXT:MX1 baseline test to assess your current level of fitness and determine your starting point.

FXT:FIT Baseline Testing

The FXT:FIT program is a prerequisite for the FXT:SXP program, which is in turn required for the FXT:EXP program. In order to test your total-body conditioning, cardiovascular fitness, speed and endurance, we'll employ a pretty straightforward test that you should use every eight weeks (see "Re-Evaluate" on page 36) to assess your progress.

The "Hot Circuit" test measures your ability to perform four exercises (pull-ups, squats, push-ups and crunches) and run, walk or jog

First-timers can skip the test! If you're looking to drop some weight and get into fitness, we make it as easy as possible to get off on the right foot and get comfortable with a simple-to-follow program. We created the FXT:PX1 program (see page 71) for you to hop right in and get going on your fitness journey (after talking to your doctor, of course). Once you've completed that program, you should be ready to take the FXT:FIT or FXT:MX1 test to see if you're ready to start either of those programs.

200 yards (less than ⅛ mile) in 20 minutes or less.

What? You want me to do all these exercises back to back? I can't do as many push-ups after my upper body is tired from pull-ups! Squats and running in the same routine? You guys are nuts.

Yes, that's the whole idea. But not that we're nuts—that you'll be performing each exercise back to back with little or no rest in between. Strength, coordination, proper form... it all starts now.

Throughout all of the fitness, speed, endurance and weight-loss programs, you'll be performing different intervals at varying intensities, so it's a good idea to see where you stand early! If you're unsure about tackling these exercises by yourself, why not invite a friend to take on this challenge with you? Having a training partner is a great way to keep you safe, motivated and accountable for your workouts. If you have a training partner for the initial test, have them keep an eye on your form to make sure you're performing the movement properly. If you're having problems with your form, now is the easiest time to fix it.

Always take the test at your own pace; rest, recover, rehydrate and refocus as needed.

Not interested in taking the test quite yet? Then use FXT:PX1 on page 71 instead of taking this rather intensive test right now. Trust us, you're better off learning the ropes and progressing through the program than jumping into the deep end before you've learned how to swim.

TAKING THE TEST

Before beginning the test, it's imperative that you prepare yourself for the exercises by warming up and getting your blood pumping. A good warm-up should be 5–10 minutes and raise your body temperature to a light sweat. Flip to page 166 for some ideas.

Here's what you'll need for the test:

Stopwatch or mobile app with timer.

Pull-up bar: Use an appropriate pull-bar that's high enough that you can extend your arms fully when grasping it. If it's too high, you may feel uncomfortable jumping up to grab it. If it's too low, you'll waste energy bending your knees to keep your feet from touching the ground. The bar itself should be safe and sturdy and able to hold more than double your body weight.
Note: Playground bars work great!

Water: Hydrate before, after and even during if you need it.

Towel: Make sure your hands are dry when performing pull-ups or push-ups so you don't slip.

Exercise mat (preferred, but optional).

Space: Your workout area should be well-ventilated and free from obstructions so you can complete the movements freely without hitting anything. Performing this test outside works best, but you can

"Hot Circuit" sprang into life as a training drill we devised to race each other and challenge ourselves to better our fitness while we were training for long-distance triathlons in 2009. The "Hot" moniker comes from our training conditions in Phoenix during summer—most days the sports complex we used was over 100 scorching degrees.

use a treadmill if your workout needs to be indoors. Be extremely careful when stepping on and off the treadmill, especially if the belt is moving!

Warmed up and ready? Great! Just a few minutes more and you can start the test. Before you do, it's very important that you familiarize yourself with the proper form of each exercise. Read each of the exercise descriptions, view the photos and slowly try each move yourself a few times to make sure you understand exactly what you'll be doing once you get started.

Make sure you're hydrated, somewhat relaxed and take some slow, deep breaths to prepare. We're starting with an exercise that's daunting for some—the pull-up. Even if you've never been able to do a pull-up in the past, it's important that you try. We've personally witnessed many people who thought they couldn't do any do three or four once they realize the proper form and use the large muscles of their upper back to complete the movement. Don't mentally block yourself from success; give it your best shot.

With each of the exercises, complete as many reps as you can, taking rest breaks as needed. If you can't complete the reps, remember how many you've completed and move on to the next portion. In order to get an accurate baseline, add :30 to your time for every repetition you failed to complete.

Example: Completed 8 pull-ups; add 1:00 to your finishing time.

Start your timer (or click "Begin Test" on the FXT:FIT mobile app) and perform:

- 10 Pull-Ups
- Run, Jog or Walk 50 yards as fast as you can
- 20 Bodyweight Squats
- Run, Jog or Walk 50 yards as fast as you can
- 20 Push-Ups
- Run, Jog or Walk 50 yards as fast as you can
- 20 Crunches
- Run, Jog or Walk 50 yards as fast as you can

Stop your timer, note the time and add any additional time from missed reps. Compare your time to the chart below.

DETERMINING YOUR LEVEL

9:59 or less

Start with FXT:FIT Advanced Level, starting on page 77

10:00–19:59

Start with FXT:FIT Basic Level, on page 77

Over 20:00

Start with the FXT:PX1, starting on page 71

Please note: If you were unable to complete any reps on any exercise, it's recommended that you start with FXT:PX1. For a large percentage of readers, pull-ups will be the deciding factor. It's important that you build them up or you'll be missing a huge part of the program.

> **TIP:** Take a "before" picture. Actually, take several from different angles. Guys, take your shirt off and, ladies, pick that bikini that you'd love to look great in. This is a really important step that's often forgotten and best taken care of before you even take the test. Personally, we wish we had some good shirt-off "before" pictures of ourselves. Truth be told, we never took any shirtless pictures because we were unhappy with the way we looked. Now we wish we had those photos to compare—and you will too! You don't need to share them with anyone else right now if you're self-conscious, but we've had trainees post them on their fridge to remind them of why they were working so hard to get fit. Keep track of your progress with a picture each week; you'll be amazed at your transformation!

FXT:MX1 Baseline Testing

Completion of the FXT:MX1 program is a prerequisite for beginning the FXT:ST1 program. Both the FXT:MX1 and FXT:ST1 programs share the same baseline test since we're simply trying to determine if you can lift the baseline numbers for the core exercises. Over the course of a week, use four separate days to work your way up to a weight that's fairly challenging, a weight you estimate would be between your 1RM (1-rep maximum), 3RM or even 5RM. The reason we include both 3RM and 5RM is that we're not huge fans of the 1RM outside of powerlifting competitions. In our view, they don't serve much purpose and open you up to injury. If you're an experienced lifter and are used to pushing to a 1RM, feel free. If not, go for a 3RM or 5RM. If you know your 3RM or 5RM, you can also use any of a number of online calculators to estimate your 1RM.

With your 1RM in hand, look at the table below. The requirements are based on your body weight and the amount you can lift in your 1RM on a particular exercise. They are:

Squat: 1.5 x your body weight

Deadlift: 2 x your body weight

Bench Press: 1.25 x body weight

Overhead Press: .75 x body weight

EXERCISE	Your weight 150lb	Your weight 200lb
Squat	225lb	300lb
Deadlift	300lb	400lb
Bench Press	187.5lb	200lb
Overhead Press	112.5lb	150lb

If your 1RM is within shouting distance of the requirements for your body weight, you have a good baseline of strength and musculature to start either FXT:MX1 or FXT:ST1 without caveat.

However, if your numbers are significantly lower than those requirements, it simply means you'll need to spend some time building a baseline of strength and muscle before moving on to more advanced programs.

SHARE YOUR SUCCESS & GET SOCIAL!

Got the FXT:FIT App? You can grab it at fxtfit.com and click away on the "Before" photo and post your progress. We've created a Facebook page for our fans to share photos, goals, successes and challenges at http://facebook.com/fxtfit. Upload your before, during and after photos to inspire yourself and others, and share your FXT Scores in the social community to constantly find new motivation, tips and techniques.

Using the FXT Point System

The point system is about as straightforward as it gets. Each workout has a Basic and Advanced Target for FXT Points and Time. Your goal is to complete the required sets at or below the Target Time. After your workout, add up all your points and you have a FXT Score to track your progress and share with your friends online.

Based on your age, weight, current physical conditioning, and your short- or long-term goals, you'll have a FXT Point Target to hit with each workout. Simply add up all the points after completing your routine to make sure you're on track with your workouts.

Target Time & Target Weight Percentage

Whether you're using one of the programs or creating your own from the 100+ exercises in this book, you'll choose the intensity based on how rapidly you can complete the workout with proper form in each exercise in relation to the Target Time and the heaviness of the weights (if required) in relation to a percentage of your body weight. Think of Target Points like scoring in golf: Whether you par, bogey or birdie a hole, you'll still continue and finish all 18 holes, right? To continue the golf metaphor, any seasoned golfer knows that it takes tons of practice to master the proper form and technique and then string it all together from stroke to stroke in order to play a sub-par round. Well, these workouts are no different. As you continue to practice form and develop total-body strength and fitness, you'll raise your intensity and thereby lower your times; as you get stronger, you'll progressively increase your weights and complete more sets to accrue more FXT Points per workout, week, month… you get the idea!

Reading the Workout Charts

FXT:FIT Day 1, Week 1
Basic Target Points: 80
Target Time: 16:00

FXT TERMS

SET: One circuit of that workout's exercises with the desired repetitions (reps).

TARGET POINTS: Essentially, how many sets you'll complete based on your goals and fitness level. We provide Basic and Advanced Target Points, and you're free to create your own as well.

TARGET TIME: A baseline for how long each workout should take at moderate intensity. Completing a workout below the target time threshold indicates a higher-intensity workout. Write your finish time in the workout log and add a "+" after your FXT Points when you share your workout with others.

DURATION/INTENSITY: Based on Target Time, the shorter the duration, the higher the intensity.

TARGET WEIGHT PERCENTAGE: This is a guideline for how much weight (barbell, dumbbell, medicine ball, etc.) you should be lifting or pushing based on your own body weight. If you weigh 150 pounds, a 50% Target Weight for an exercise would be 75 pounds.

Note: Target Weight Percentage is a guideline—use only weights that allow you to perform all the reps of a given exercise with proper form. Start light and increase as you progress through the programs. Not all exercises require weights.

FXT SCORE: Add up all the FXT Points for sets completed during your workout and note the duration; give a "+" or "-" for intensity. Example: 80+ FXT Score

Advanced Target Points: 120
Target Time: 18:00
Instructions: Complete as many sets as possible with good form. Rest as needed.

- 20 Bodyweight Squats (5 points)
- 1:00 Plank (5 Points)
- 20 Lunges (5 Points)
- 20 Push-Ups (5 Points)

FXT Score: Completing (4) sets of the above equals 80; (5) sets total 100.

Completing desired rounds above or below target time indicates intensity; add "+" for below, "-" for above. Example: 80+ FXT Score

FXT:MX1 Day 1, Week 1

Basic Target Points: 100

Advanced Target Points: 140

Instructions: Complete as many sets as possible with good form. Rest as needed.

- 10 Ball Thrusters (5 Points)
- 10/side One-Arm Rows (5 Points)
- 10 Pull-Ups (5 Points)
- 20 Push-Ups (5 Points)

FXT Score: Completing (5) sets of the above program will yield 100 FXT Points (Basic Target met); (7) sets equals 140 points (Advanced Target met).

Completing desired rounds above or below target time indicates intensity; add "+" for below, "-" for above. Example: 100- FXT Score

Note: FXT:MX1 and FXT:ST1 do not have a Target Time, as both of these workouts have required time under tension and are designed to be performed while focusing on form rather than completion time. See the chart on page 62 for guidelines on how much weight you should be targeting based on a percentage of your body weight.

What Intensity Means to Your Workout

Possibly the biggest mistake and the most potential for injury is not knowing how much you should do. Don't listen to anything other than your body here! Don't listen to your buddy, some random guy in the gym, a trainer or, most importantly, your ego. Let it all go. Listen to your body.

Intensity is individual. We, Brett and Jason, are built very differently. If Brett tried to lift as much as Jason in the gym for the squat, it's a one-way ticket to snap city. If Jason tried to run as fast for as far as Brett, he'd be getting his post-run smoothie intravenously in the ER.

The key to intensity is that it, along with the programs, is always changing and progressive. If you try to bench press 200 pounds on day one, you're just being stupid. But day 90? You might be able to! Heck, day 90 might have you doing 250 pounds for reps. Similarly, don't try to run 12 miles off the bat—work up to that. Intensity is about knowing your individual limits, flirting with them on a daily basis and blowing through them through smart training, proper nutrition and adequate recovery. FXT's not about vanity or ego. It's about developing athletic prowess, strength, speed, endurance and, most of all, lifelong fitness. Follow the plans, progress and make it a habit to train on the edge of your limits without going over them.

With the caveats out of the way, intensity is CRITICAL to all the programs. If you're not continually challenging yourself, you aren't progressing. We can't stress this enough. How many times have you seen someone in the gym lifting the exact same weight they were lifting a year ago? Are they vastly physically different than they were a year ago? If someone runs the same distance at the same pace year-round, is their marathon time improving? Nope. It's less about the time you put in and more about the quality of that time.

Frankly, what's more de-motivating than spending countless hours "training" to not see improvement? The quickest way to not achieve your goals is to quit trying. And the secret to sticking with it is looking past today to tomorrow, when you know you'll be better than

you were today because of the effort you put in. Trust us—any momentary discomfort during the training session itself is well worth the reward as you progress. Keep it up. Keep pushing. Stick with it and don't let up. Trust the process. Tomorrow you'll be better off than today. Next week you'll be better than this week. Next year you'll be a whole new you.

Exertion Scale

When performing the workouts, your intensity is directly tied to your results and is determined by your duration of exercise, force applied and exertion. Here are the quick definitions of perceived exertion based on ability to hold a conversation, and obviously these are relative to the fitness and conditioning of each individual and will change as you become fitter.

EASY: You should be able to carry on a conversation and breathe relatively normally. An easy pace is good for warm-up, cool-down, recovery the day or two after a hard-run race, or running long distances. Easy runs or jogs are roughly 40–65% of your maximal effort.

MODERATE: Your breathing should be faster than normal due to your elevated heart rate and exertion. While you can't carry on a full conversation, you can speak in occasional sentences. Moderate, or tempo, runs help to build strength and endurance. Moderate runs are about 65–85% of your maximal effort.

HARD: This is all-out sprinting. You'll be breathing extremely hard and unable to speak more than a word or so at a time. Hard intervals are done for a short period of time to build speed and train fast-twitch muscle fibers to respond even when fatigued. Hard runs represent over 85% of your maximal effort.

TARGET HEART RATE & ZONES

If you're a bit more attuned to data and happen to own a heart monitor (or like to do math), you can use the following Attainable Heart Rate equation to calculate your Target Heart Rate (THR). *Note:* This is not exact and can fluctuate by as much as 15 beats per minute (BPM); use this only as a guideline (100% = maximal effort).

$$220 - AGE \times ZONE\% = THR$$

ZONE 1 (EASY):
40–65%—WARM-UP & COOL-DOWN/RECOVERY

ZONE 2 (MODERATE):
65%–85%—AEROBIC ENDURANCE

ZONE 3 (HARD):
85%—PEAK ZONE/ANAEROBIC THRESHOLD

For example, a 30-year-old male looking for his Target Heart Rate (THR) at a 70% effort has a THR of 133 BPM:

$$220 - 30 \times 70\% = 133$$

Whether you use perceived exertion level or heart rate zones to calculate your intensity, it's important to listen to your body and also to follow the guidelines in the workouts. An easy effort shouldn't be at high intensity, and there's a good chance you shouldn't be chatting up your running partner during extremely hard, intense workouts.

How Long Should My Program Be?

Over the last few years, we've gotten this question quite a bit by e-mail and during interviews: "What's with the whole '7 Weeks' thing in all your books and how did you come up with it?" General sports and fitness training for events is a year-round event for a lot of people (us included), and it's extremely necessary to change your routine every so often to avoid plateaus, overtraining, and mental or physical burnout. Even professional athletes take a good chunk of their off-season to engage in different sports or activities and change their workout routines.

Guess what? Seven to eight weeks is the optimal window for learning a new routine, adapting to the exercises and the new demands on your body, perfecting the form and reaping the benefits, and then testing yourself. This can be a running or obstacle race, setting a new 1-rep max, looking in the mirror or checking how your clothes are fitting. From there, you'll re-evaluate your routine or goals and then make some simple modifications to you program's points through added intensity, weight or duration.

WEEK 1: Learn the routine. Everyone's a beginner once—don't rush through this part or you'll knock yourself off-track with delayed onset muscle soreness (DOMS) by overdoing it too quickly. Take your time and learn the exercises and proper form by performing them slowly and carefully. This will pay off come week 3 or so.

WEEKS 1–3: Adapt to the exercises, working through initial soreness and making the training a part of your routine. This actually starts with your first or second workout. Some athletes take 10–14 days, while others need 18–21 to lock it in. During this period, 50 percent of workouts fail because individuals don't rearrange their lives a little bit to make the new program work. Life happens, but you can always come back and pick up here or start over.

WEEKS 3–8: Perfect the form. This is the sweet spot and the reason why you took it slow on week 1 and stuck with it—you'll be seeing the most strength and fitness gains. There will be one or more times during this 28-day period where you feel bulletproof. Remember, you may be a rockstar, but you're not made of Kevlar. Act accordingly.

WEEK 8: Re-evaluate your program, rest, recover and adapt your program to fit new goals. Whether you're using this book for fat loss, body shaping or sport-specific training, you can transition to and from each of the goal-based workouts in this book to others rather easily. Since this is cross-training program, you should keep running and exercising. Just take it down a notch and allow for some rest and recovery. This is similar to the run-specific term "taper"; the exercise version is called a "deload" week. You'll be performing a lighter workload for the next seven days until you start up a new program or modify your existing one with added points or intensity. It'll provide the exercise to keep you loose, but a reduced workload to allow you to recover, reset and plan the next goal for you to dominate.

FXT:PX1
Intro to FXT

Welcome to FXT:PX1, the Intro to FXT program. More importantly, welcome to the beginning of your fitness lifestyle journey! Whether you're looking to prepare for the FXT:FIT or the FXT:MX1 programs, FXT:PX1 is an awesome opportunity for men and women of all fitness levels to build the full-body strength they'll need to become fitter, faster and stronger athletes.

The main goal of this program is to provide an easy, controlled method for learning proper form for some of the most important exercises for total-body fitness without having to worry about a certain number of reps or sets. Think of FXT:PX1 as the foundation that you'll build your fitness lifestyle upon—you wouldn't rush and build a cheap foundation for your house, right? FXT:PX1 allows you to build up your strength and endurance progressively over eight weeks while learning proper form for 10 exercises (plus variations) and developing your own unique fitness lifestyle routine that fits into your daily life.

We realize you're learning new exercises and movements, adapting to a whole new exercise and nutrition routine, and actually performing the fitness training all at the same time, and we all know that it isn't easy. If it takes you eight weeks or eight months to get fit, it's still well worth the effort!

This is also as good a time as any to bring up the topic of weight (specifically body fat) loss, as it's one of the most common questions we get via e-mail from all over the world and a huge part of developing the physique you're working for. In Part Four, we have an entire section on fueling the athlete (see page 169).

Here are some tips that will help you make the most of your program:

- DO NOT overdo any workouts, especially the first couple of weeks! You WILL be sore for one or two days after your first few workouts, and if you overdo by attempting to do too many reps too quickly, you'll miss subsequent workouts. This happens to nearly everyone when they start a workout regimen—don't let it happen to you. If you haven't exercised in quite some time, then take the first week or two extra easy and work your way up.

- Follow the nutritional advice consistent with the FXT:FIT plan (page 77) to make sure you have the energy and nutrients needed to perform the workouts, recover, and rebuild your muscles.

- Stick with it! You'll always miss some workouts, no matter how hard you try and prepare—life gets in the way. Don't be discouraged if you miss a day—just pick up immediately where you left off. If you missed a week, just restart the following Monday. Don't give up. The goal is all about you getting in the best shape of your life. Even if it takes eight months of stops and starts, with some perseverance and tenacity you'll meet your goals.

If you're planning to move up to FXT:MX1, we recommend using the weighted and plyometric variations to build muscle and strength to prepare you for the demands of that program. See "FXT:MX1 Prep: Plyometric & Weighted Variations" (page 73).

Getting Started with FXT:PX1

This program is built around exercising 20 minutes a day, 5 days a week. For some individuals who are exercising for the first time or coming back after a long layoff, start with at least one week of exercising for a maximum of 10 minutes. Three of those days you'll be walking, jogging or running at your own pace, which means you may walk 19:30 and jog for :30 if you're fresh off the couch. Seasoned runners may jog all 20 minutes. Either way, you're getting the right workout relative to your own ability. The other two days you'll be performing as many sets of bodyweight exercises as you can while using proper form. You control the number of sets, intensity and rest between exercises or sets. It's all relative to your ability, and all up to you.

FXT:PX1 TARGETS

While we provide a baseline FXT Points Target (60/25 FXT Points), each week, you should be striving to increase your performance by 10% in number of reps or distance. See the examples below:

EXERCISES

- **Week 1:** Complete 1 set in 20:00; your goal for Week 2 is to complete your first set at least 1:00–2:00 faster.

- **Week 1:** Cover 1 mile in 20:00; your Week 2 goal should be to increase your distance between 1.1 and 1.2 miles.

FXT:PX1 POINTS KEY

10 Reps of bodyweight exercises	= 2.5	Points
1 min walk/jog	= 3	Points
1 min for moderate intensity running	= 5	Points
1 min for high intensity (sprint, hill repeats, etc.)	= 7	Points

FXT:MX1 PREP: PLYOMETRIC & WEIGHTED VERSIONS

Are you looking to progress to the FXT:MX1 program or use FXT:PX1 to build some more muscle? Utilizing the weighted or plyometric variations of the standard FXT:PX1 exercises can surely help. We recommend completing the entire eight-week FXT:PX1 program and focusing on good form and making progressive improvements before utilizing these more difficult and demanding variations.

FXT:PX1 EXERCISE	PLYOMETRIC OR WEIGHTED VARIATIONS
Squat *(page 148)*	Jump Squat, Medicine Ball, or Dumbbell Goblet Squat
Hip Raise *(page 141)*	Hip Thruster
Flutter Kick *(page 134)*	Flutter Kick with ankle weights
Superman *(page 131)*	Superman with wrist weights, light dumbbells or medicine ball
Push-Up *(page 156)*	Clapping Push-Up
Reverse Crunch *(page 139)*	Reverse Crunch with ankle weights or medicine ball clasped between feet
Bird Dog *(page 137)*	Bird Dog with ankle & wrist weights
Mountain Climber *(page 144)*	Mountain Climber with ankle & wrist weights
Lunge *(page 150)*	Jump Lunge, lunge while holding a medicine ball
Marching Twist *(page 142)*	Marching Twist holding medicine ball

FXT:PX1 Program

Warm up for 5 minutes prior to each workout; stretch after completion. Warm-Ups & Stretches start on page 166.

Week 1

DAY 1		
Exercise	Distance/ Reps	Points
20:00 Walk/Jog Intervals (60 FXT Points)		
DAY 2		
20:00 as many sets as possible		
10 Squat (2.5 FXT Points) *p. 148*		
10 Hip Raise (2.5 FXT Points) *p. 141*		
10 Flutter Kick (2.5 FXT Points) *p. 134*		
10 Superman (2.5 FXT Points) *p. 131*		
10 Push-Up (2.5 FXT Points) *p. 156*		
DAY 3		
20:00 Walk/Jog Intervals (60 FXT Points)		
DAY 4		
20:00 as many sets as possible		
10 Reverse Crunch (2.5 FXT Points) *p. 139*		
10 Bird Dog (2.5 FXT Points) *p. 137*		
10 Cobra (2.5 FXT Points) *p. 131*		
10 Lunge (2.5 FXT Points) *p. 150*		
10 Marching Twist (2.5 FXT Points) *p. 142*		
DAY 5		
20:00 Walk/Jog Intervals (60 FXT Points)		
DAY 6		
Rest		
DAY 7		
Rest		

Week 2

DAY 1		
Exercise	Distance/ Reps	Points
20:00 Walk/Jog Intervals (60 FXT Points)		
DAY 2		
20:00 as many sets as possible		
10 Squat (2.5 FXT Points) *p. 148*		
10 Hip Raise (2.5 FXT Points) *p. 141*		
10 Flutter Kick (2.5 FXT Points) *p. 134*		
10 Superman (2.5 FXT Points) *p. 131*		
10 Push-Up (2.5 FXT Points) *p. 156*		
DAY 3		
20:00 Walk/Jog Intervals (60 FXT Points)		
DAY 4		
20:00 as many sets as possible		
10 Reverse Crunch (2.5 FXT Points) *p. 139*		
10 Bird Dog (2.5 FXT Points) *p. 137*		
10 Cobra (2.5 FXT Points) *p. 131*		
10 Lunge (2.5 FXT Points) *p. 150*		
10 Marching Twist (2.5 FXT Points) *p. 142*		
DAY 5		
20:00 Walk/Jog Intervals (60 FXT Points)		
DAY 6		
Rest		
DAY 7		
Rest		

Week 3

DAY 1		
Exercise	Distance/ Reps	Points
20:00 Walk/Jog Intervals (60 FXT Points)		
DAY 2		
20:00 as many sets as possible		
10 Squat (2.5 FXT Points) p. 148		
10 Hip Raise (2.5 FXT Points) p. 141		
10 Flutter Kick (2.5 FXT Points) p. 134		
10 Superman (2.5 FXT Points) p. 131		
10 Push-Up (2.5 FXT Points) p. 156		
DAY 3		
20:00 Walk/Jog Intervals (60 FXT Points)		
DAY 4		
20:00 as many sets as possible		
10 Reverse Crunch (2.5 FXT Points) p. 139		
10 Bird Dog (2.5 FXT Points) p. 137		
10 Cobra (2.5 FXT Points) p. 131		
10 Lunge (2.5 FXT Points) p. 150		
10 Marching Twist (2.5 FXT Points) p. 142		
DAY 5		
20:00 Walk/Jog Intervals (60 FXT Points)		
DAY 6		
Rest		
DAY 7		
Rest		

Week 4

DAY 1		
Exercise	Distance/ Reps	Points
20:00 Walk/Jog Intervals (60 FXT Points)		
DAY 2		
20:00 as many sets as possible		
10 Squat (2.5 FXT Points) p. 148		
10 Hip Raise (2.5 FXT Points) p. 141		
10 Flutter Kick (2.5 FXT Points) p. 134		
10 Superman (2.5 FXT Points) p. 131		
10 Push-Up (2.5 FXT Points) p. 156		
DAY 3		
20:00 Walk/Jog Intervals (60 FXT Points)		
DAY 4		
20:00 as many sets as possible		
10 Reverse Crunch (2.5 FXT Points) p. 139		
10 Bird Dog (2.5 FXT Points) p. 137		
10 Cobra (2.5 FXT Points) p. 131		
10 Lunge (2.5 FXT Points) p. 150		
10 Marching Twist (2.5 FXT Points) p. 142		
DAY 5		
20:00 Walk/Jog Intervals (60 FXT Points)		
DAY 6		
Rest		
DAY 7		
Rest		

Success!

Congratulations on completing FXT:PX1! During the program you've learned extremely valuable lessons about developing a fitness routine and making it work with your everyday life—and that's the whole point! There's no such thing as a "quick fix" when it comes to getting our bodies fit. It requires patience and diligence to build a fitness lifestyle that works for you. As we've mentioned before, you can come back to this routine anytime and modify it with the weighted or plyometric variations or dial the intensity up or down to suit your goals.

Are you ready for the challenge of FXT:FIT or FXT:MX1? Then take the Baseline Test on page 60 and see how much progress you've made!

FXT:FIT
Total-Body Fitness & Weight Loss

What's your definition of fit? Does it involve being able to tighten your belt a notch or two, running a mile non-stop, hitting a 300-yard drive down the middle of the fairway, or seeing your abdominal muscles for the first time since you were a teenager? If your goal is to develop total-body strength, lose weight and make your physique leaner and more athletic, you've chosen the right program!

With its combination of bodyweight and weighted exercises along with high-intensity cardiovascular training, FXT:FIT is your key to building and maintaining optimal functional fitness—in other words, keeping you strong, flexible, dexterous, fast and ready to participate in nearly any athletic activity. Whether you treat this program as your "fountain of youth" to get you back into the same shape as your glory days or a first step in getting from the couch to the starting line of a 5K or mud run, the FXT:FIT is a go-to fitness routine that anyone can use anytime and nearly anywhere to tone, strengthen and condition your body.

This is a complete body program, meaning you need to perform all the exercises to develop optimum functional fitness—do not skip exercises because you don't like them or they're difficult to complete. They were specifically chosen for their effectiveness at delivering results.

In addition, finish every rep and set. Whether you're on pace to finish below the target time or double that amount, the only way you'll transform your mind and body is to develop consistency and tenacity from one workout to the next.

Essentially, prior to starting your timer and performing the first movement, commit yourself to completing the entire workout. Don't cheat your success by quitting early. Rest as needed and focus on your form—only stop when you can no longer perform each exercise properly or can no longer continue due to extreme fatigue, light-headedness, acute pain or other injury warning signs.

As we mentioned earlier in "Using the FXT Point System" on page 63, each workout has a point total that's created by the sum of the individual exercises and reps. Keeping track

Completion of the FXT:FIT program is a prerequisite for starting the FXT:SXP program. FXT:FIT will provide the foundation for the more-intense, full-body, explosive workouts you'll be using in FXT:SXP, which in turn will prepare you for the extremely intense FXT:EXP program.

of your point total is an important tool to keep your progression on track. In order to develop as an athlete, you'll have to continually set the bar a little higher from week to week and re-evaluate your entire fitness regimen every eight weeks. How do you do that? Add more weight or more reps, or complete the workout at a higher intensity in a shorter amount of time. Oh, and feel free to share your FXT Score with all your friends on social media. Even the ones who may grumble about your fitness posts are probably getting inspired by you and motivated to start working out themselves. Trust us, we've seen it hundreds of times!

Progressive Workouts

As we'll cover in the FXT:EXP section, developing a deep well of muscular endurance comes from training at a high level even when at or near muscular exhaustion. The easiest concept to hammer this home is this: You'll make more endurance and strength gains from the last 5 reps than you will from the first 5. Muscular stress builds muscle—actually, it tears muscles apart, only to regrow them stronger. If you're a runner, finishing a workout strong is akin to finishing a race with a swift "kick" as the finish line comes into view. No matter how difficult the beginning or middle of a workout is, finishing strong—and with good form—is its own reward and amplifies gains.

These progressive workout styles break from the common boredom of cranking out multiple sets with the same number of reps when you're working to build speed, endurance and total-body fitness (5x5 lifts do play a strong part in FXT:MX1 and FXT:ST1, but not here). Because each workout requires you to build up or down depending on the type you choose, you have a finite start and finish point. So finish each and every one of these workouts—unless you're light-headed, dizzy or injured, of course. The magic of these progressives is directly tied to you completing every rep, got it?

When following the progressive programs below, you'll be adding 1 rep each set, and those reps add up very quickly. For example, a "1-10 ladder" consists of 10 sets with a total of 55 reps. Yes, you read that correctly—that innocuous little "1-10" results in 55 total reps! We added a helpful chart after each progressive exercise description below to help with the math so you know what you're getting into before you start. A "10-20-10 pyramid" results in a whopping 330 reps. Yes, you read that right.

LADDERS

This multiple-set workout increases the workload incrementally from set to set, making the lifts near the end of the workout exponentially more difficult. Excellent for building strength and muscle endurance, ladders require increasing levels of effort and attention to maintain good form during the later sets. Bodyweight exercises or exercises using a light weight are recommended for this type of regimen.

Perform one additional exercise rep each set, sequentially adding more reps until the end of the workout.

Set/Rep example: Set 1, 1 rep; Set 2, 2 reps...Set 10, 10 reps

Pattern example: 1, 2, 3, 4, 5, 6, 7, 8, 9, 10

LADDER MATH

Sets	Rep Progression	Total Reps
5	1–5	15
10	1–10	55
10	5–15	110
10	10–20	165

REVERSE LADDERS

A multiple-set workout designed for maximizing metabolic and muscle stress, reverse ladders start with many repetitions at the beginning of a workout and end with very few. This structure allows athletes to complete each successive set with proper form due to the reduction in repetitions while allowing for a heavier weight to be used versus the traditional ladder, even though they both require the same number of reps.

Perform one less exercise rep per set, sequentially reducing the number of reps until the end of the workout.

Set/Rep example: Set 1, 10 reps; Set 2, 9 reps...Set 10, 1 rep

Pattern Example: 10, 9, 8, 7, 6, 5, 4, 3, 2, 1

REVERSE LADDER MATH

Sets	Rep Progression	Total Reps
5	5 –1	15
10	10 –1	55
10	15 –5	110
10	20 –10	165

PYRAMIDS

Also a multiple-set workout, pyramids start similarly to ladders with low reps and incrementally add one rep of each exercise up to the "peak" or highest point of the pyramid before reversing the trend, reducing the repetitions by one each set until reaching the original number. By starting the workout with minimal reps, pyramids provide an effective warm-up when utilizing heavy weights and then progressively build to become increasingly more difficult before eventually returning to decreasing reps.

> **Set/Rep example:** Set 1, 1 rep; Set 2, 2 reps...Set 5, 5 reps; Set 6, 5 reps...Set 10, 1 rep.
>
> **Pattern example:** 1, 2, 3, 4, 5, 5, 4, 3, 2, 1

PYRAMID MATH

Sets	Rep Progression	Total Reps
10	1–5 –1	30
10	5–10–5	90
5	10–15–10	150
10	10–20–10	330

REVERSE PYRAMIDS

The exact opposite of pyramids when it comes to addition and subtraction of reps, reverse pyramids start at the highest number of reps and decrease incrementally until the low point of reps is hit, then increase one rep per set until reaching and completing the peak number of reps again. This type of workout can be performed with relatively heavy weights, provided an adequate warm-up set is performed, and is equally suited for lighter weights or bodyweight exercises. The inverse nature of reverse pyramids is slightly more beneficial for building muscle stress and endurance versus standard pyramids, as the maximum number of reps is required at the end of the workout as muscle fatigue is setting in.

Set/Rep example: Set 1, 5 rep; Set 2, 4 reps...Set 5, 1 rep; Set 6, 1 rep...Set 10, 5 reps

Pattern example: 5, 4, 3, 2, 1, 1, 2, 3, 4, 5

REVERSE PYRAMID MATH

Sets	Rep Progression	Total Reps
10	5–1–5	30
10	10–5–10	90
5	15–10–15	150
10	2--10–20	330

SEESAWS

This workout type is a combination of ladders, reverse ladders, pyramids and reverse pyramids with two or more exercises. Just like the playground equipment this progression is named after, the seesaw drill has one side going up while the other goes down. These programs perform extremely well with one light weight or bodyweight exercise and one heavier weighted or more "technical" lift to build total-body strength and muscle endurance.

Ladder Seesaw features one exercise (generally the more technical, heavier one) starting from 1 and progressing upward to 10, while the second exercise (generally a bodyweight exercise) descends from 10 to 1.

> **Exercise 1A Pattern Example:** 1, 2, 3, 4, 5, 6, 7, 8, 9, 10 (55 total reps)
>
> **Exercise 1B Pattern Example:** 10, 9, 8, 7, 6, 5, 4, 3, 2, 1 (55 total reps)
>
> See "Ladder Math" on page 79 for other sample total reps.

Pyramid Seesaw utilizes the pyramid for one exercise (generally the more technical, heavier one) and a reverse pyramid for the second exercise (generally a bodyweight exercise). These "mirror" pyramids will always require the same number of reps split between the two exercises:

Exercise 1A Pattern Example: 1, 2, 3, 4, 5, 5, 4, 3, 2, 1 (30 total reps)

Exercise 1B Pattern Example: 5, 4, 3, 2, 1, 1, 2, 3, 4, 5 (30 total reps)

Note: In the example above, each set has 6 reps (1+5, 2+4, etc.) as you'll be alternating back and forth between exercises 1 and 2. Pretty cool, huh?

FXT Drills

A big part of the FXT:FIT, FXT:SXP and FXT:EXP programs is the high-intensity interval (HIIT) drills that are used to develop speed, strength and flexibility, as well as torch fat and keep the programs interesting, exciting and really, really intense. Always follow the instructions for warm-up and cool-down, hydrate properly and take a break if you feel light-headed or dizzy. These drills are no joke, and it's up to you to provide the intensity to make them incredibly effective at building the strength, speed and athletic performance you crave.

40S DRILL

During the NFL combine, the 40-yard sprint, or "40 time," is crucial for assessing how highly players will be drafted, and quite literally is worth millions of dollars in salary to these athletes. While these 40s will make you faster and stronger, they won't necessarily be capable of padding your bank account with a seven-figure paycheck. But hey, money can't buy fitness, strength and endurance! Just like the NFL combine, you'll want to time your effort and continually strive toward finishing in faster and faster times.

This drill can be performed with 10–30 seconds of rest after each sprint and exercise. Eventually you should progress to complete this workout without any rest.

40-yard sprint

10 push-ups

40-yard sprint

10 jumping lunges

40-yard sprint

10 burpees

40-yard sprint

10 air squats

40-yard sprint

30 crunches

That's one rep. Hydrate and rest as necessary before repeating!

HOT CIRCUIT 2 DRILL

The original "Hot Circuit" that we created back in 2008 is used as the FXT:FIT test on page 59. This version is slightly different and a little more challenging. The layout still works perfectly on a football field, soccer pitch or any 100-yard-by-50-yard flat patch of grass. Perform each sprint/mobility exercise and bodyweight exercise as a circuit, resting only when absolutely necessary. Eventually, you should progress to completing this entire workout without resting, then take a quick break, sip of water and repeat. It's called "Hot Circuit" for a reason; it'll burn fat right off of your body!

Remember to use a timer, and progressively chop down the amount of time it takes you to complete each round.

10 push-ups

50-yard backward sprint

20 in & outs

25-yard sprint

25-yard walking lunges

10 narrow push-ups

50-yard crab walk

10 wide push-ups

50-yard burpee jumps

50 jumping jacks

12.5-yard inchworm

25-yard bear crawl

12.5-yard spiderman

30 marching twists

50-yard sprint

10 push-ups

BURPEE MILE DRILL

This ridiculous challenge came from Mike DeAngelo, our close friend and trainer, who wanted to really push his limits. Start out by linking 5 or 10 burpee jumps (see description below) together and continually add distance as you progress. MikeyD completed the full mile (5280 feet) on his first attempt in 1:16:28 and approximately 1550 burpee jumps (he totally lost count—I bet you can figure out why!).

MikeyD's top-3 tips:

- Wear gloves.

- Use a deep squat and a big arm swing to build up the force to jump as far as possible. The farther you jump, the fewer burpees you'll need to do!

- Wear a hat or something to drop and mark your spot if you need to leave your spot when nature calls.

Burpee jumps are a plyometric move that start out as a traditional burpee (the "full version" including the push-up) and incorporate an arm swing toward the back and an explosive two-legged broad jump forward as far as possible, followed by a controlled landing.

1. Stand tall with your back erect, feet shoulder-width apart and toes rotated slightly outward.

2. Shift your hips backward and sit back for the squat, keeping your head up and bending your knees. Lean your weight forward and place your hands on the floor inside, outside or in front of your feet—whichever is more comfortable and gives you a nice, stable base.

3. Kick your feet straight back so that you're now in a push-up start position, forming a straight line from your head to your feet. Keep your core tight to maintain an erect spine.

4. Inhale as you lower your torso toward the floor for a push-up. Stop when your body is 1–2 inches from the floor.

5. Exhaling, straighten your arms and propel your entire upper body off the floor while simultaneously bending your knees and bringing them toward your chest in order to plant your feet underneath you. You should end up back in the bottom position of a squat. Take a quick breath.

6. Swing your arms down and behind you in an arc, then reverse your arm direction forward, exhale and explode forward in a broad jump from the toes of both feet. Land with your knees slightly bent to absorb the impact.

That's 1 rep.

REVOLUTIONS DRILL

Find a running track at a school or park and develop speed, explosive power and endurance with this combination of traditional running drills and plyometric moves. This routine is all about intensity and leg mobility; you'll be running the 800-yard sections exceptionally hard (after a warm-up, of course) and performing the plyometric moves with explosive force. If Revolutions don't have you sucking wind after one rep, you're not pushing yourself hard enough!

800 yards

40 Striders

40 Butt Kicks

40 High Knees

40 Skips

800 yards

That's 1 rep. Rest 10 to 60 seconds, hydrate and repeat.

Nutrition to Get FIT

There's a good amount of truth to the adage "You are what you eat," and for this book we'll modify the phrase to focus on eating for performance: "Your engine needs fuel to run." On page 169 we cover the necessary micro- and macro-nutrients required to keep an athlete fueled for training and primed for recovery and growth.

FXT:FIT POINTS KEY

20 Bodyweight Reps	=	5 FXT points	Ladders, Pyramids, sequential drills	=	5 FXT points /10 Reps
10 Weighted Reps	=	5 FXT points	Hot Circuit 2	=	50 FXT points/round
Walk/Jog	=	3 FXT points/min	Revolutions	=	50 FXT points/round
Moderate Run	=	5 FXT points/min	40s Drill	=	20 FXT points/round
Hard Run/Sprint	=	7 FXT points/min			

Add up all your points to get your FXT Score.

INTENSITY:

If you finish above or below the Target Time, append the amount of time that you exceed over the Target Time to the end of your score.

Example: 20:00 Target Time, 22:00 finish = +2:00

EXAMPLE:

Basic Target Points: 80, Target Time: 16:00

Advanced Target Points: 120, Target Time: 18:00

Instructions: Complete as many sets as possible with good form. Rest as needed.

20 Bodyweight Squats = 5 points

1:00 Plank = 5 points

20 Lunges = 5 points

(20) Push-Ups = 5 points

Example: Completed 4 sets of the above in 20:00.

Score: 80 +4:00

FXT:FIT Program

Warm up for 5 minutes prior to each workout; stretch after completion. Warm-Ups & Stretches start on page 166. Use exertion scale on page 67 for Easy, Moderate and Hard effort. Complete as many reps as possible with good form to reach Target Points & Target Time.

Week 1

DAY 1

TARGET POINTS *Basic:* 80   *Advanced:* 120
TARGET TIME   *Basic:* 16:00   *Advanced:* 18:00

Exercise	Reps / Pts	Rounds	Time	Pts Total
Squat *p. 148*	20 / 5			
1:00 Plank *p. 136*	1:00 / 5			
Lunge *p. 150*	20 / 5			
Push-Up *p. 156*	20 / 5			

Basic: 4x; *Advanced:* 5x

DAY 2

TARGET POINTS *Basic:* 60   *Advanced:* 100
TARGET TIME   *Basic:* 20:00   *Advanced:* 20:00

Exercise	Reps / Pts	Rounds	Time	Pts Total
20:00 Jog/Run Intervals *or* 20:00 Walk/Jog Intervals				

Basic: Easy Run; *Advanced:* Moderate Run

DAY 3

TARGET POINTS *Basic:* 80   *Advanced:* 120
TARGET TIME   *Basic:* 16:00   *Advanced:* 18:00

Exercise	Reps / Pts	Rounds	Time	Pts Total
Mason Twist *p. 133*	20 / 5			
Hip Raise *p. 141*	20 / 5			
Side Plank *p. 137*	:30 per side / 5			
Inchworm *p. 137*	10 / 2.5			
Superman *p. 131*	10 / 2.5			

Basic: 4x; *Advanced:* 5x

Week 2

DAY 1

TARGET POINTS *Basic:* 80   *Advanced:* 120
TARGET TIME   *Basic:* 16:00   *Advanced:* 18:00

Exercise	Reps / Pts	Rounds	Time	Pts Total
Marching Twist *p. 142*	20 / 5			
Hanging Leg Raise *p. 141*	10 / 2.5			
Lunge *p. 150*	20 / 5			
Push-Up *p. 156*	20 / 5			
Mountain Climber *p. 144*	10 / 2.5			

Basic: 4x; *Advanced:* 5x

DAY 2

TARGET POINTS *Basic:* 60   *Advanced:* 100
TARGET TIME   *Basic:* 20:00   *Advanced:* 20:00

Exercise	Reps / Pts	Rounds	Time	Pts Total
20:00 Jog/Run Intervals				

Basic: Easy Run; *Advanced:* Moderate Run

DAY 3

TARGET POINTS *Basic:* 80   *Advanced:* 120
TARGET TIME   *Basic:* 16:00   *Advanced:* 18:00

Exercise	Reps / Pts	Rounds	Time	Pts Total
Weighted Hip Thrust *p. 141*	20/5			
Burpee *p. 144*	20/5			
Swoop & Touch *p. 131*	1:00/5			
Goblet Squat *p. 148*	20/5			

Basic: 4x; *Advanced:* 5x

FXT:FIT Program

Warm up for 5 minutes prior to each workout; stretch after completion. Warm-Ups & Stretches start on page 166. Use exertion scale on page 67 for Easy, Moderate and Hard effort. Complete as many reps as possible with good form to reach Target Points & Target Time.

Week 3

DAY 1

TARGET POINTS *Basic:* 80   *Advanced:* 120
TARGET TIME   *Basic:* 16:00   *Advanced:* 18:00

Exercise	Reps / Pts	Rounds	Time	Pts Total
Ball Thruster p. 147	10 / 5			
Wall Ball p. 147	10 / 2.5			
Jump Lunge p. 150	10 / 2.5			
Push-Up p. 156	20 / 5			
Dip p. 160	10 / 2.5			

Basic: 4x; *Advanced:* 5x

DAY 2

TARGET POINTS *Basic:* 75   *Advanced:* 125
TARGET TIME   *Basic:* 25:00   *Advanced:* 25:00

Exercise	Reps / Pts	Rounds	Time	Pts Total
25:00 Jog/Run Intervals				

Basic: Easy Run; *Advanced:* Tempo Run

DAY 3

TARGET POINTS *Basic:* 80   *Advanced:* 120
TARGET TIME   *Basic:* 16:00   *Advanced:* 18:00

Exercise	Reps / Pts	Rounds	Time	Pts Total
Weighted Hip Thrust p. 141	10 / 5			
Burpee p. 144	20 / 5			
Plank p. 136	1:00 / 5			
Pull-Up p. 156	10 / 2.5			
Side Plank Fly p. 139	10 / 2.5			

Basic: 4x; *Advanced:* 5x

Week 4

DAY 1

TARGET POINTS *Basic:* 80   *Advanced:* 120
TARGET TIME   *Basic:* 16:00   *Advanced:* 18:00

Exercise	Reps / Pts	Rounds	Time	Pts Total
Pull-Up p. 156	10 / 2.5			
Triceps Kickback p. 160	10 per side / 5			
Burpee p. 144	20 / 5			
V-Sit p. 132	20 / 5			
Dip p. 160	10 / 2.5			

Basic: 4x; *Advanced:* 5x

DAY 2

TARGET POINTS *Basic:* 80   *Advanced:* 100
TARGET TIME   *Basic:* 20:00   *Advanced:* 20:00

Exercise	Reps / Pts	Rounds	Time	Pts Total
10:00 Jump Rope p. 165 Basic, Skier, Bell				
10:00 Jog/Run Intervals				

Basic: Easy Run; *Advanced:* Pick-up Run

DAY 3

TARGET POINTS *Basic:* 80   *Advanced:* 120
TARGET TIME   *Basic:* 16:00   *Advanced:* 18:00

Exercise	Reps / Pts	Rounds	Time	Pts Total
Single-Arm Curl & Press p. 157	10 per side / 5			
Linear Reactive Step-Up p. 154	10 per side / 5			
Side Plank p. 137	:30 per side / 5			
Reverse Fly p. 162	10 / 2.5			
Inchworm p. 137	10 / 2.5			

Basic: 4x; *Advanced:* 5x

FXT:FIT Program

Warm up for 5 minutes prior to each workout; stretch after completion. Warm-Ups & Stretches start on page 166. Use exertion scale on page 67 for Easy, Moderate and Hard effort. Complete as many reps as possible with good form to reach Target Points & Target Time.

Week 5

DAY 1

TARGET POINTS *Basic:* 80   *Advanced:* 120
TARGET TIME   *Basic:* 16:00   *Advanced:* 18:00

Exercise	Reps / Pts	Rounds	Time	Pts Total
Lunge with Twist *p. 151*	10 per side / 5			
Med Ball Burpee *p. 144*	10 / 5			
Ab Crunch/Toe Touch *p. 132*	10 / 5			
Turkish Get-Up *p. 135*	5 / 2.5			
Med Ball Good Morning *p. 152*	5 / 2.5			

Basic: 4x; *Advanced:* 5x

DAY 2

TARGET POINTS *Basic:* 50   *Advanced:* 100
TARGET TIME   *Basic:* 15:00   *Advanced:* 22:00

Exercise	Reps / Pts	Rounds	Time	Pts Total
Marching Twist *p. 142*	20 / 5			
Jump Rope Basic *p. 165*	1:00 / 5			
Skier *p. 165*	1:00 / 5			
Bell *p. 165*	1:00 / 5			
Side Hop *p. 143*	20 / 5			

Basic: 2x; *Advanced:* 4x

DAY 3

TARGET POINTS *Basic:* 60   *Advanced:* 90
TARGET TIME   *Basic:* 14:00   *Advanced:* 16:00

Exercise	Reps / Pts	Rounds	Time	Pts Total
Burpee *p. 144*	20 / 5			
Lunge with Biceps Curl *p. 151*	10 per side / 5			
Bird Dog *p. 137*	10 / 2.5			
Hip Raise *p. 141*	10 / 2.5			

Basic: 4x; *Advanced:* 5x

Week 6

DAY 1

TARGET POINTS *Basic:* 80   *Advanced:* 120
TARGET TIME   *Basic:* 16:00   *Advanced:* 18:00

Exercise	Reps / Pts	Rounds	Time	Pts Total
Lunge with Twist *p. 151*	10 per side / 5			
Single-Leg Squat *p. 149*	10 per side / 5			
Ab Crunch/Toe Touch *p. 132*	10 / 5			
Hanging Leg Raise *p. 141*	10 / 2.5			
Mountain Climbers *p. 144*	10 / 2.5			

Basic: 4x; *Advanced:* 5x

DAY 2

TARGET POINTS *Basic:* 100   *Advanced:* 140
TARGET TIME   *Basic:* 15:00   *Advanced:* 22:00

Exercise	Reps / Pts	Rounds	Time	Pts Total
Plank Row *p. 139*	10 per side / 5			
Wood Chop *p. 134*	20 / 5			
Reverse Crunch *p. 139*	20 / 5			
Superman *p. 131*	10 / 2.5			
Hip Raise *p. 141*	10 / 2.5			

Basic: 5x; *Advanced:* 7x

DAY 3

TARGET POINTS *Basic:* 80   *Advanced:* 120
TARGET TIME   *Basic:* 16:00   *Advanced:* 18:00

Exercise	Reps / Pts	Rounds	Time	Pts Total
Skater Hop *p. 143*	10 per side / 5			
Goblet Squat *p. 148*	10 / 5			
Step-Up w/DB Curl *p. 155*	10 per side / 5			
Dip *p. 160*	20 / 5			

Basic: 4x; *Advanced:* 5x

FXT:FIT Program

Warm up for 5 minutes prior to each workout; stretch after completion. Warm-Ups & Stretches start on page 166. Use exertion scale on page 67 for Easy, Moderate and Hard effort. Complete as many reps as possible with good form to reach Target Points & Target Time.

Week 7

DAY 1

TARGET POINTS *Basic:* 45   *Advanced:* 75
TARGET TIME   *Basic:* 18:00   *Advanced:* 24:00

Exercise	Reps / Pts	Rounds	Time	Pts Total
Ladder: Deadlift *p. 152*	1-5 / 7.5			
Ladder: Pull-Up *p. 156*	1-5 / 7.5			

Basic: 3x; *Advanced:* 5x

DAY 2

TARGET POINTS *Basic:* 60   *Advanced:* 120
TARGET TIME   *Basic:* 20:00   *Advanced:* 32:00

Exercise	Reps / Pts	Rounds	Time	Pts Total
40s Drill	1 / 20			

Basic: 3x; *Advanced:* 6x

DAY 3

TARGET POINTS *Basic:* 60   *Advanced:* 120
TARGET TIME   *Basic:* 14:00   *Advanced:* 20:00

Exercise	Reps / Pts	Rounds	Time	Pts Total
Pyramid Seesaw: **1A** = Pyramid; **1B** = Reverse Pyramid				
1A: Landmine *p. 163*	5-1-5 / 15			
1B: Overhead Press *p. 157*	1-5-1 / 15			

Basic: 2x; *Advanced:* 4x

Week 8

DAY 1

TARGET POINTS *Basic:* 90   *Advanced:* 135
TARGET TIME   *Basic:* 16:00   *Advanced:* 22:00

Exercise	Reps / Pts	Rounds	Time	Pts Total
Pyramid Seesaw: **1A** = Pyramid; **1B** = Reverse Pyramid				
1A: Burpee with Overhead Press and Lunge *p. 145*	5-1-5 / 15			
1B: Push-Up *p. 156*	1-5-1 / 15			
1B: In & Out *p. 131*	1-5-1 / 15			

Basic: 2x; *Advanced:* 3x

DAY 2

TARGET POINTS *Basic:* 50   *Advanced:* 100
TARGET TIME   *Basic:* 20:00   *Advanced:* 32:00

Exercise	Reps / Pts	Rounds	Time	Pts Total
Hot Circuit 2 *p. 81*	1 / 50			

Basic: 1x; *Advanced:* 2x

DAY 3

TARGET POINTS *Basic:* 60   *Advanced:* 120
TARGET TIME   *Basic:* 14:00   *Advanced:* 20:00

Exercise	Reps / Pts	Rounds	Time	Pts Total
Pyramid Seesaw: **1A** = Pyramid; **1B** = Reverse Pyramid				
1A: Clean *p. 153*	5-1-5 / 15			
1B: Pull-Up *p. 156*	1-5-1 / 15			

Basic: 2x; *Advanced:* 4x

Success!

Congratulations on completing the FXT:FIT program! You've engaged in one of the most comprehensive total-body functional fitness programs available and taken your athletic ability to new heights—but don't stop yet! Each FXT program, whether it's the FIT, Strength, Muscle, Speed, Endurance and even Intro to FXT program, was designed to be a program that you can use over and over to continue to develop strength, speed, muscle, endurance and a healthy, active body. Just because you've completed one round of one specific program doesn't in any way mean you should disregard it and move on! You can always improve your results relative to target points and time— add more weight to your reps and perform each and every exercise with perfect form to enhance your fitness and shred your physique. Of course, we're absolutely encouraging you to mix it up and try out all the different programs in the book as they fit your goals over time. The entire nature of cross training is to switch up your workout at regular intervals to develop all your musculature at multiple disciplines on a range of different planes—not just focus on specific muscles by continually training a set range of motion with the same exercises. To steal a line from one of Brett's favorite movies of all time, *Fight Club:* "I say evolve, and let the chips fall where they may."

FXT:SXP
Developing Explosive Speed & Athletic Performance

Congratulations again on finishing the FXT:FIT program, and welcome to the next step to improving your strength, speed, flexibility and fitness. FXT:SXP is pretty extreme and built to challenge athletes of all levels because the level of intensity that you put into every rep of every exercise and every single drill is controlled by you.

If you're not totally spent near the end of each workout, you're not pushing yourself hard enough nor setting the groundwork to smash the plateaus of "fatigue" or "exhaustion" that limit your ability now. Developing explosive speed is about finding the next gear and blowing past your current thresholds and trouncing your current levels of athletic performance. Whether your goal is a faster 40-yard time, crushing a new 5K personal record or playing for longer then ever at a higher level at team sports like soccer, football or basketball, FXT:SXP is the place to start.

In the SXP program we'll focus on strengthening your legs, trunk and core with easy-to-follow exercises, develop your fast-twitch muscles and explosive power using plyometrics, and use mobility and flexibility drills to develop your overall speed. On top of all that, we'll even do some running. This is an intense regimen with some high-tempo plyometric moves and elements from the FXT:FIT complete-body program. Prior to starting your timer and performing the first movement, commit yourself to completing the entire workout. Don't cheat your success by quitting early. Rest as needed and focus on your form—only stop when you can no longer perform each exercise properly or can no longer continue due to extreme fatigue, light-headedness, acute pain or other injury warning signs.

You'll need to perform all the exercises to develop optimum functional fitness—do not skip exercises because you don't like them or they're difficult to complete. They were specifically chosen for their effectiveness at delivering results. In addition, finish every rep and set. Whether you're on pace to finish below the target time or double that amount, the only

FXT:FIT is a prerequisite for FXT:SXP. Completion of FXT:SXP is required before starting FXT:EXP. Your mantra for this program should be: "Run when you can, walk if you have to, crawl if you must; just never give up" (Dean Karnazes).

way you'll transform your mind and body is to develop consistency and tenacity from one workout to the next. Developing speed requires performing some exercises and drills at high intensity, but not all of them. You can't push your body 100% all the time, so follow the routine, including tempo and pace, and observe the proper rest periods.

Speed Drills

Pop quiz: What's the quickest way to develop explosive speed? Running, running and more running, right?

Of course you need to work on your running in order to develop stronger leg, hip and glute muscles, but you also need to strengthen those muscles with cross-training and implement some plyometric moves to develop your fast-twitch muscle fibers. What you may not realize is that the most important muscles you need to develop to run quickly or for long periods of time are not located in your legs, but your core. Yeah, we already covered your hips and glutes, but your abs, obliques, intercostals and erector spinae (lower back) muscles need to be strong and flexible to allow you to run quickly and efficiently.

The following drills have been designed to develop explosive power through plyometric movements, increase your foot speed through high turnover exercises and increase your flexibility by extending your range of motion.

THE 20/20 DRILL

The 20/20 Drill combines eight moves at high intensity to develop your speed, strength, agility, endurance and all-around athletic ability. This drill is short and intense as a workout, and also provides a great warm-up and cool-down when performed at a more relaxed pace.

The set-up is simple: Find a flat area at least 20 yards long and place some cones or markers at each end; pavement or grass is fine, but a sports field is optimal. Perform the first exercise/movement for 20 yards until you reach your marker, turn around, and perform the next exercise/movement 20 yards back to the starting point, continually progressing through all eight moves at a high intensity, with good form and little to no rest in between.

High Knees: Run forward using a normal-length stride. Bend the knee of your elevated leg 90 degrees and raise it until it's level with your waist. Push forward from the ball of your grounded foot. Pump your arms to generate leg drive and speed. Switch legs and repeat.

Butt Kicks: Run forward by taking very small steps and raising the heel of your back leg up toward your butt. Push forward from the ball of your grounded foot, progressing 12 to 18 inches per stride.

Striders: Bound forward by pushing off hard from the ball of your grounded foot, pumping your arms to generate leg drive and speed. Take huge leaps forward, trying to cover as much ground as possible with each stride.

Skips: Bound forward by pushing off hard from the ball of your grounded foot, landing again on that same foot, and pushing off once more before landing on the opposite foot. Pump your arms to generate leg drive and speed. Take smaller leaps forward than when performing Striders, covering slightly less ground per stride.

Side Shuffle: Turn sideways with your left hip pointing toward the direction you'll be traveling, feet slightly wider than your shoulders and hands at your sides. Push off with your right foot in the direction you'll be traveling while lifting your left foot and swinging your right foot toward the center of your body. Touch both feet together lightly before landing on your right foot, extending your left foot out to the side in the direction you're traveling and repeating the process. When you reach the halfway point (the 10-yard mark), turn 180 degrees so that your right hip is pointing in the direction that you're traveling and continue side shuffling an additional 10 yards.

Walking Lunge: Stand tall, facing the direction you'll be traveling, with your feet shoulder-width apart and your arms hanging at your sides. Take a large step forward with your right foot, bend both knees, and drop your hips straight down until both knees are bent 90 degrees. Your left knee should almost be touching the ground and your left toes are on the ground behind you. Keep your core engaged and your back, neck and hips straight at all times during this movement. Keeping your right foot in place on the ground, push up with your right leg, straighten both knees, bring your left leg parallel with your right, and place your left foot next to your right. Continue moving forward by repeating the above process with your left foot.

Backward Sprint: Facing away from the direction you'll traveling, run by pushing off alternating forefeet and raising your knees as high as possible. Pump your arms as needed to generate leg drive and speed. This takes a little getting used to but it's a great way to strengthen your running muscles by working them in an opposite plane of motion and helps to develop balance and agility.

Sprint: The sprint is saved for last so you're working extremely hard to generate speed after your legs and lungs are already fatigued. Run forward at top speed by leaning forward with your upper body to as much as a 45-degree angle and driving off the balls of your feet as hard and as rapidly as you can. Pump your arms to increase leg drive and speed.

HILL REPEATS

Hill repeats develop leg strength through the added force needed to combat gravity while climbing an incline. They also change the angle of each footfall and push-off to work muscles in a new range of motion.

First, you'll need a paved hill that's long enough for you to run up for at least 20 seconds, or up to 100 strides. A straight sidewalk, long driveway or safe side road will do. The hill doesn't need to be very steep (at least when you're just getting started) but should be enough of a bump to make a 20-second sprint up it a bit of a chore. Avoid grass, trails or stairs unless absolutely necessary as the focus of this drill is to build your running strength without having to focus on your footing, obstacles or tripping over a step. Even if you're training for a trail race, this is a smooth-surface exercise; you can get your trail practice during your weekly mileage outside of these drills. Need to use a treadmill? See below.

The intervals are performed by running up the hill at the chosen level of exertion for the designed amount of time or number of strides. Once you hit that goal, slow, stop and turn around to descend the hill for the next repeat; this may be a walk or a slow jog to return to the start position. Don't dilly-dally, however— get back to the start for your next interval as quickly as you can while catching your breath. Hill repeats are quick, brutal and effective—the quicker you get them over with, the sooner you can re-hydrate and move on with your workout.

Treadmill users: While you'll be missing out on the downhill walk or jog with each repetition, you can effectively use the treadmill to dial in a speed and incline that suits your athletic ability and goals. Follow the appropriate warm-up of 5 minutes with the incline set at .5 or 1% and then carefully grab the handrails and step on the side rails while raising the incline to 5–10% based on your ability; change the speed so that you can safely maintain a moderate pace for the desired time. You'll need to adjust the incline and speed settings to hit your targets, so don't be afraid to carefully step off the belt if needed and make changes. When performing the intervals, run at the desired speed for the amount of time or strides in the program and then carefully step off the belt onto the side rails to rest. Since you won't be walking or jogging downhill, take a 30-second to 1-minute break before your next interval, unless specifically instructed in the chart.

PICK-UPS

Understanding pick-up intervals is pretty easy; performing them is slightly more difficult. After warming up, you'll run for the specified distance or time at a designated pace or exertion level and then—you guessed it—"pick up" your speed for an interval of time. Once your faster interval is over, return back to the previous pace or exertion level and continue. You may drop your intensity all the way down to a walk for 30 seconds or so if you need to catch your breath, hydrate and recover.

Treadmill users should have no problem with this—just crank up the speed for the desired amount of time. The speed increase is relative to your ability and goals.

TEMPO RUNS

Tempo runs are easily defined as running for a prescribed period of time at a "hard" exertion level, or above 85% of your maximal effort or target heart rate (see "Total Heart Rate & Zones" on page 68). Once again, this pace is relative to your ability and as you progress it's a moving target. Keep that in mind when another runner shares their tempo pace or tries to tell you that it should be ANY exact minutes

per mile. Your tempo is your tempo and it will change from month to month based on your training. Got it?

Nutrition for Speed & Explosive Performance

Nutrition plays a big part in fueling for training and getting the long-term body composition you want. Refer to "Nutrition for FXT:FIT, FXT:SXP & FXT:EXP on page 174 for guidelines on meal timing and macro- and micronutrient consumption. You'll also learn how what you take in before, during and after training affects your success.

FXT:SXP POINTS KEY

20 Bodyweight Reps	= 5 FXT Points		Ladders, Pyramids, sequential drills	= 5 FXT Points /10 Reps
10 Weighted Reps	= 5 FXT Points		Hot Circuit 2	= 50 FXT Points/round
Walk/Jog	= 3 FXT Points/min		Revolutions	= 50 FXT Points/round
Moderate Run	= 5 FXT Points/min		40s Drill	= 20 FXT Points/round
Hard Run/Sprint	= 7 FXT Points/min			

Add up all your points to get your FXT Score.

INTENSITY:

If you finish above or below the Target Time, append the amount of time that you exceed over the Target Time to the end of your score.

Example: 20:00 Target Time, 22:00 finish = +2:00

EXAMPLE:

Basic Target Points: 80, Target Time: 16:00

Advanced Target Points: 120, Target Time: 18:00

Instructions: Complete as many sets as possible with good form. Rest as needed.

20 Bodyweight Squats = 5 points

1:00 Plank = 5 points

20 Lunges = 5 points

(20) Push-Ups = 5 points

Example: Completed 4 sets of the above in 20:00.

Score: 80 +4:00

FXT:SXP Program | Week 1

Warm up for 5 minutes prior to each workout; stretch after completion. Warm-Ups & Stretches start on page 166. Use exertion scale on page 67 for Easy, Moderate and Hard effort. Complete as many reps as possible with good form to reach Target Points & Target Time.

DAY 1

TARGET POINTS *Basic:* 60   *Advanced:* 90
TARGET TIME   *Basic:* 20:00   *Advanced:* 24:00

Exercise	Reps / Pts	Rounds	Time	Pts Total
1-Mile Run (1:00-2:00 Walk as needed)				

Basic: Easy Run, repeat 2x
Advanced: Moderate Run, repeat 3x

DAY 2

TARGET POINTS *Basic:* 40   *Advanced:* 80
TARGET TIME   *Basic:* 15:00   *Advanced:* 23:00

Exercise	Reps / Pts	Rounds	Time	Pts Total
Jumping Jacks *p. 142*	20 / 5			
Push-Up *p. 156*	20 / 5			
Mountain Climber *p. 144*	20 / 5			
Lunge *p. 150*	20 / 5			

Basic: 2x; *Advanced:* 4x

DAY 3

TARGET POINTS *Basic:* 60   Advanced: 90
TARGET TIME   *Basic:* 20:00   Advanced: 24:00

Exercise	Reps / Pts	Rounds	Time	Pts Total
1-Mile Run				

Basic: Easy Run, repeat 2x
Advanced: Moderate Run, repeat 3x

DAY 4

TARGET POINTS *Basic:* 40   *Advanced:* 80
TARGET TIME   *Basic:* 15:00   *Advanced:* 23:00

Exercise	Reps / Pts	Rounds	Time	Pts Total
Mason Twist *p. 133*	20 / 5			
Hip Raise *p. 141*	20 / 5			
Superman *p. 131*	20 / 5			
Plank *p. 136*	1:00 / 5			

Basic: 2x; *Advanced:* 4x

DAY 5

TARGET POINTS *Basic:* 60   *Advanced:* 90
TARGET TIME   *Basic:* 20:00   *Advanced:* 24:00

Exercise	Reps / Pts	Rounds	Time	Pts Total
1-Mile Run				

Basic: Easy Run, repeat 2x
Advanced: Moderate Run, repeat 3x

DAY 6

Rest

DAY 7

TARGET POINTS *Basic:* 75   *Advanced:* 125
TARGET TIME   *Basic:* 25:00   *Advanced:* 25:00

Exercise	Reps / Pts	Rounds	Time	Pts Total
Walk/Jog/Run				

Basic: Easy Run; *Advanced:* Moderate Run

FXT:SXP Program | Week 2

Warm up for 5 minutes prior to each workout; stretch after completion. Warm-Ups & Stretches start on page 166. Use exertion scale on page 67 for Easy, Moderate and Hard effort. Complete as many reps as possible with good form to reach Target Points & Target Time.

DAY 1

TARGET POINTS *Basic:* 60   *Advanced:* 90
TARGET TIME   *Basic:* 20:00   *Advanced:* 24:00

Exercise	Reps / Pts	Rounds	Time	Pts Total
1-Mile Run				

Basic: Easy Run, repeat 2x
Advanced: Moderate Run, repeat 3x

DAY 2

TARGET POINTS *Basic:* 40   *Advanced:* 80
TARGET TIME   *Basic:* 18:00   *Advanced:* 25:00

Exercise	Reps / Pts	Rounds	Time	Pts Total
Marching Twist p. 142	20 / 5			
Squat p. 148	20 / 5			
Wood Chop p. 134	20 / 5			
Inchworm p. 137	10 / 2.5			
Push-Up p. 156	10 / 2.5			

Basic: 2x; *Advanced:* 4x

DAY 3

TARGET POINTS *Basic:* 50   *Advanced:* 100
TARGET TIME   *Basic:* 20:00   *Advanced:* 32:00

Exercise	Reps / Pts	Rounds	Time	Pts Total
Hot Circuit 2 p. 81	1 / 50			

Basic: 1x; *Advanced:* 2x

DAY 4

TARGET POINTS *Basic:* 40   *Advanced:* 80
TARGET TIME   *Basic:* 15:00   *Advanced:* 23:00

Exercise	Reps / Pts	Rounds	Time	Pts Total
Side Plank p. 137	:30 per side / 5			
Hip Raise p. 141	20 / 5			
In & Out p. 131	20 / 5			
Flutter Kick p. 134	20 / 5			

Basic: 2x; *Advanced:* 4x

DAY 5

TARGET POINTS *Basic:* 60   *Advanced:* 90
TARGET TIME   *Basic:* 20:00   *Advanced:* 24:00

Exercise	Reps / Pts	Rounds	Time	Pts Total
1-Mile Run				

Basic: Easy Run, repeat 2x
Advanced: Moderate Run, repeat 3x

DAY 6

Rest

DAY 7

TARGET POINTS *Basic:* 75   *Advanced:* 125
TARGET TIME   *Basic:* 25:00   *Advanced:* 25:00

Exercise	Reps / Pts	Rounds	Time	Pts Total
Walk/Jog/Run				

Basic: Easy Run; *Advanced:* Moderate Run

FXT:SXP Program | Week 3

Warm up for 5 minutes prior to each workout; stretch after completion. Warm-Ups & Stretches start on page 166. Use exertion scale on page 67 for Easy, Moderate and Hard effort. Complete as many reps as possible with good form to reach Target Points & Target Time.

DAY 1

TARGET POINTS *Basic:* 90   *Advanced:* 120
TARGET TIME   *Basic:* 30:00   *Advanced:* 32:00

Exercise	Reps / Pts	Rounds	Time	Pts Total
1-Mile Run				

Basic: Easy Run, repeat 2x
Advanced: Moderate Run, repeat 3x

DAY 2

TARGET POINTS *Basic:* 70   *Advanced:* 105
TARGET TIME   *Basic:* 22:00   *Advanced:* 24:00

Exercise	Reps / Pts	Rounds	Time	Pts Total
Box Jump *p. 155*	20 / 5			
Lunge *p. 151*	20 / 5			
Mountain Climber *p. 144*	20 / 5			
Mason Twist *p. 133*	10 / 2.5			
Side Plank *p. 137*	:30 per side / 5			
Superman *p. 131*	20 / 5			
Bicycle Crunch *p. 138*	20 / 5			

Basic: 2x; *Advanced:* 3x

DAY 3

TARGET POINTS *Basic:* 50   *Advanced:* 100
TARGET TIME   *Basic:* 20:00   *Advanced:* 32:00

Exercise	Reps / Pts	Rounds	Time	Pts Total
20/20 Drill *p. 91*	1 / 20			

Basic: 1x; *Advanced:* 2x

DAY 4

TARGET POINTS *Basic:* 110   *Advanced:* 140
TARGET TIME   *Basic:* 30:00   *Advanced:* 34:00

Exercise	Reps / Pts	Rounds	Time	Pts Total
10:00 Jump Rope Basic *p. 165*	1 / 50			
Skier *p. 165*	1 / 50			
Bell *p. 165*	1 / 50			
1-Mile Run				

Basic: Easy Run, repeat 2x
Advanced: Moderate Run, repeat 4x

DAY 5

TARGET POINTS *Basic:* 60   *Advanced:* 120
TARGET TIME   *Basic:* 20:00   *Advanced:* 32:00

Exercise	Reps / Pts	Rounds	Time	Pts Total
40s Drill *p. 81*	1 / 20			
1 Mile Run				

Basic: Easy Run, repeat 2x
Advanced: Moderate Run, repeat 3x

DAY 6

Rest

DAY 7

TARGET POINTS *Basic:* 105   *Advanced:* 175
TARGET TIME   *Basic:* 35:00   *Advanced:* 35:00

Exercise	Reps / Pts	Rounds	Time	Pts Total
Walk/Jog/Run				

Basic: Easy Run; *Advanced:* Moderate Run

FXT:SXP Program | Week 4

Warm up for 5 minutes prior to each workout; stretch after completion. Warm-Ups & Stretches start on page 166. Use exertion scale on page 67 for Easy, Moderate and Hard effort. Complete as many reps as possible with good form to reach Target Points & Target Time.

DAY 1

TARGET POINTS *Basic:* 90   *Advanced:* 120
TARGET TIME   *Basic:* 30:00   *Advanced:* 32:00

Exercise	Reps / Pts	Rounds	Time	Pts Total
1-Mile Run				

Basic: Easy Run, repeat 3x
Advanced: Moderate Run, repeat 4x

DAY 2

TARGET POINTS *Basic:* 60   *Advanced:* 80
TARGET TIME   *Basic:* 24:00   *Advanced:* 32:00

Exercise	Reps / Pts	Rounds	Time	Pts Total
Burpee *p. 144*	20 / 5			
T-Twist *p. 133*	20 / 5			
Bird Dog *p. 137*	10 / 2.5			
Hip Raise *p. 141*	10 / 2.5			
Box Jump *p. 155*	20 / 5			

Basic: 3x; *Advanced:* 4x

DAY 3

TARGET POINTS *Basic:* 50   *Advanced:* 100
TARGET TIME   *Basic:* 20:00   *Advanced:* 32:00

Exercise	Reps / Pts	Rounds	Time	Pts Total
Hill repeats :20 Moderate :30 Walk/Rest :20 Hard :30 Walk/Rest	1 / 10			

Basic: 5x; *Advanced:* 10x

DAY 4

TARGET POINTS *Basic:* 70   *Advanced:* 105
TARGET TIME   *Basic:* 22:00   *Advanced:* 24:00

Exercise	Reps / Pts	Rounds	Time	Pts Total
Box Jump *p. 155*	20 / 5			
Lunge *p. 150*	20 / 5			
Mountain Climber *p. 144*	20 / 5			
Mason Twist *p. 133*	20 / 5			
Side Plank *p. 137*	:30 per side			
Superman *p. 131*	20 / 5			
Bicycle Crunch *p. 138*	20 / 5			

Basic: 2x; *Advanced:* 3x

DAY 5

TARGET POINTS *Basic:* 90   *Advanced:* 120
TARGET TIME   *Basic:* 30:00   *Advanced:* 32:00

Exercise	Reps/ Points	Rounds	Time	Pts Total
1-Mile Run				

Basic: Easy Run, repeat 3x
Advanced: Moderate Run, repeat 4x

DAY 6

Rest

DAY 7

TARGET POINTS *Basic:* 135   *Advanced:* 225
TARGET TIME   *Basic:* 45:00   *Advanced:* 45:00

Exercise	Reps / Pts	Rounds	Time	Pts Total
Walk/Jog/Run				

Basic: Easy Run; *Advanced:* Moderate Run

FXT:SXP Program | Week 5

Warm up for 5 minutes prior to each workout; stretch after completion. Warm-Ups & Stretches start on page 166. Use exertion scale on page 67 for Easy, Moderate and Hard effort. Complete as many reps as possible with good form to reach Target Points & Target Time.

DAY 1

TARGET POINTS *Basic:* 90   *Advanced:* 120
TARGET TIME   *Basic:* 30:00   *Advanced:* 32:00

Exercise	Reps / Pts	Rounds	Time	Pts Total
1-Mile Run				

Basic: Easy Run, repeat 3x
Advanced: Moderate Run, repeat 4x

DAY 2

TARGET POINTS *Basic:* 60   *Advanced:* 120
TARGET TIME   *Basic:* 14:00   *Advanced:* 20:00

Exercise	Reps / Pts	Rounds	Time	Pts Total
Pyramid Seesaw: **1A** = Pyramid; **1B** = Reverse Pyramid				
1A: Landmine *p. 163*	1-5-1 / 15			
1B: Overhead Press *p. 157*	5-1-5 / 15			

Basic: 2x; *Advanced:* 4x

DAY 3

TARGET POINTS *Basic:* 40   *Advanced:* 80
TARGET TIME   *Basic:* 18:00   *Advanced:* 25:00

Exercise	Reps / Pts	Rounds	Time	Pts Total
20/20 Drill *p. 91*	1 / 20			

Basic: 2x; *Advanced:* 4x

DAY 4

TARGET POINTS *Basic:* 70   *Advanced:* 105
TARGET TIME   *Basic:* 22:00   *Advanced:* 24:00

Exercise	Reps / Pts	Rounds	Time	Pts Total
Single-Leg Deadlift *p. 153*	20 / 5			
Jump Lunge *p. 150*	20 / 5			
Mountain Climber *p. 144*	20 / 5			
Mason Twist *p. 133*	20 / 5			
Side Plank *p. 137*	:30 per side / 5			
Superman *p. 131*	20 / 5			
Bicycle Crunch *p. 138*	20 / 5			

Basic: 2x; *Advanced:* 3x

DAY 5

TARGET POINTS *Basic:* 90   *Advanced:* 120
TARGET TIME   *Basic:* 30:00   *Advanced:* 32:00

Exercise	Reps / Pts	Rounds	Time	Pts Total
1-Mile Run				

Basic: Easy Run, repeat 3x
Advanced: Moderate Run, repeat 4x

DAY 6

Rest

DAY 7

TARGET POINTS *Basic:* 150   *Advanced:* 225
TARGET TIME   *Basic:* 50:00   *Advanced:* 45:00

Exercise	Reps / Pts	Rounds	Time	Pts Total
5-Mile Run				

Basic: Easy Run; *Advanced:* Moderate Run

FXT:SXP Program | Week 6

Warm up for 5 minutes prior to each workout; stretch after completion. Warm-Ups & Stretches start on page 166. Use exertion scale on page 67 for Easy, Moderate and Hard effort. Complete as many reps as possible with good form to reach Target Points & Target Time.

DAY 1

TARGET POINTS *Basic:* 90   *Advanced:* 120
TARGET TIME   *Basic:* 30:00   *Advanced:* 32:00

Exercise	Reps / Pts	Rounds	Time	Pts Total
1-Mile Run				

Basic: Easy Run, repeat 3x
Advanced: Moderate Run, repeat 4x

DAY 2

TARGET POINTS *Basic:* 120   *Advanced:* 240
TARGET TIME   *Basic:* 18:00   *Advanced:* 22:00

Exercise	Reps / Pts	Rounds	Time	Pts Total
Pyramid Seesaw: **1A** = Pyramid; **1B** = Reverse Pyramid				
1A: Overhead Press with Triceps Extension *p. 158*	5-1-5 / 15			
1A: Ball Thruster *p. 147*	5-1-5 / 15			
1B: Push-Up *p. 156*	5–1–5 / 15			
1B: In & Out *p. 131*	1-5-1 / 15			

Basic: 2x; *Advanced:* 4x

DAY 3

TARGET POINTS *Basic:* 150   *Advanced:* 165
TARGET TIME   *Basic:* 27:00   *Advanced:* 21:00

Exercise	Reps / Pts	Rounds	Time	Pts Total
1-Mile Run				

Basic: Moderate Run, repeat 3x
Advanced: Hard Run, repeat 3x

DAY 4

TARGET POINTS *Basic:* 60   *Advanced:* 80
TARGET TIME   *Basic:* 24:00   *Advanced:* 32:00

Exercise	Reps / Pts	Rounds	Time	Pts Total
Burpee *p. 144*	20 / 5			
Bizarro Burpee *p. 145*	20 / 5			
Bird Dog *p. 137*	10 / 2.5			
Hip Raise *p. 141*	10 / 2.5			
Box Jump *p. 155*	:30 per side / 5			

Basic: 3x; *Advanced:* 4x

DAY 5

TARGET POINTS *Basic:* 90   *Advanced:* 120
TARGET TIME   *Basic:* 30:00   *Advanced:* 32:00

Exercise	Reps / Pts	Rounds	Time	Pts Total
1-Mile Run				

Basic: Easy Run, repeat 3x
Advanced: Moderate Run, repeat 4x

DAY 6

Rest

DAY 7

TARGET POINTS *Basic:* 70   *Advanced:* 105
TARGET TIME   *Basic:* 23:00   *Advanced:* 19:00

Exercise	Reps / Pts	Rounds	Time	Pts Total
6-Mile Run				

Basic: Easy Run; *Advanced:* Moderate Run

FXT:SXP Program | Week 7

Warm up for 5 minutes prior to each workout; stretch after completion. Warm-Ups & Stretches start on page 166. Use exertion scale on page 67 for Easy, Moderate and Hard effort. Complete as many reps as possible with good form to reach Target Points & Target Time.

DAY 1

TARGET POINTS *Basic:* 90   *Advanced:* 120
TARGET TIME   *Basic:* 40:00   *Advanced:* 40:00

Exercise	Reps / Pts	Rounds	Time	Pts Total
1-Mile Run				

Basic: Easy Run, repeat 4x
Advanced: Moderate Run, repeat 5x

DAY 2

TARGET POINTS *Basic:* 50   *Advanced:* 100
TARGET TIME   *Basic:* 20:00   *Advanced:* 32:00

Exercise	Reps / Pts	Rounds	Time	Pts Total
Hot Circuit 2 *p. 81*	1 / 50			

Basic: 1x; *Advanced:* 2x

DAY 3

TARGET POINTS *Basic:* 135   *Advanced:* 150
TARGET TIME   *Basic:* 27:00   *Advanced:* 21:00

Exercise	Reps / Pts	Rounds	Time	Pts Total
1-Mile Run				

Basic: Moderate Run, repeat 3x
Advanced: Hard Run, repeat 3x

DAY 4

TARGET POINTS *Basic:* 45   *Advanced:* 60
TARGET TIME   *Basic:* 18:00   *Advanced:* 22:00

Exercise	Reps / Pts	Rounds	Time	Pts Total
Ladder Seesaw: **1A** = Ladder; **1B** = Reverse Ladder				
1A: Deadlift *p. 152*	1-5 / 7.5			
1B: Pull-Up *p. 156*	5-1 / 7.5			

Basic: 3x; *Advanced:* 4x

DAY 5

TARGET POINTS *Basic:* 110   *Advanced:* 170
TARGET TIME   *Basic:* 35:00   *Advanced:* 28:00

Exercise	Reps / Pts	Rounds	Time	Pts Total
1 Mile Run 1:00 Rest				
Plank *p. 136*	1:00 / 5			
Hip Raise *p. 141*	20 / 5			
In & Out *p. 131*	20 / 5			
Flutter Kick *p. 134*	20 / 5			

Basic: 3x; *Advanced:* 4x

DAY 6

Rest

DAY 7

TARGET POINTS *Basic:* 70   *Advanced:* 105
TARGET TIME   *Basic:* 23:00   *Advanced:* 19:00

Exercise	Reps / Pts	Rounds	Time	Pts Total
6.2-Mile Run				

Basic: Easy Run; *Advanced:* Moderate Run

FXT:SXP Program | Week 8

Warm up for 5 minutes prior to each workout; stretch after completion. Warm-Ups & Stretches start on page 166. Use exertion scale on page 67 for Easy, Moderate and Hard effort. Complete as many reps as possible with good form to reach Target Points & Target Time.

DAY 1

TARGET POINTS *Basic:* 90   *Advanced:* 120
TARGET TIME   *Basic:* 40:00   *Advanced:* 40:00

Exercise	Reps / Pts	Rounds	Time	Pts Total
1-Mile Run				

Basic: Easy Run, repeat 4x
Advanced: Moderate Run, repeat 5x

DAY 2

TARGET POINTS *Basic:* 80   *Advanced:* 120
TARGET TIME   *Basic:* 20:00   *Advanced:* 32:00

Exercise	Reps / Pts	Rounds	Time	Pts Total
40s Drill *p. 81*	1 / 20			

Basic. 4x; *Advanced.* 6x

DAY 3

TARGET POINTS *Basic:* 80   *Advanced:* 120
TARGET TIME   *Basic:* 20:00   *Advanced:* 32:00

Exercise	Reps / Pts	Rounds	Time	Pts Total
1-Mile Run	1 / 20			

Basic: Moderate Run, repeat 3x
Advanced: Hard Run, repeat 3x

DAY 4

TARGET POINTS *Basic:* 120   *Advanced:* 180
TARGET TIME   *Basic:* 16:00   *Advanced:* 22:00

Exercise	Reps / Pts	Rounds	Time	Pts Total
Pyramid Seesaw: **1A** = Reverse Pyramid; **1B** = Pyramid				
1A: Stability Ball Extension *p. 140*	5-1-5 / 15			
1A: Ball Thruster *p. 147*	5-1-5 / 15			
1B: Push-Up *p. 156*	1-5-1 / 15			
1B: In & Out *p. 131*	1-5-1 / 15			

Basic: 2x; *Advanced:* 3x

DAY 5

TARGET POINTS *Basic:* 110   *Advanced:* 170
TARGET TIME   *Basic:* 35:00   *Advanced:* 28:00

Exercise	Reps / Pts	Rounds	Time	Pts Total
3-Mile Run 1:00 Rest				
Plank *p. 136*	1:00 / 5			
Hip Raise *p. 141*	20 / 5			
Elephant Twist *p. 134*	10 per side / 5			
Flutter Kick *p. 134*	20 / 5			

DAY 6

Rest

DAY 7

TARGET POINTS *Basic:* 70   *Advanced:* 105
TARGET TIME   *Basic:* 23:00   *Advanced:* 19:00

Exercise	Reps / Pts	Rounds	Time	Pts Total
6.2-Mile Run				

Basic: Easy Run; *Advanced:* Moderate Run

Success!

Congratulations on completing the SXP program! Take a good, long look in the mirror as not only should you be proud of what you've accomplished, the image staring back at you should be leaner, stronger and faster. Whether your goal is a new personal record in a 5K or 10K, your newfound strength, flexibility, durability and speed will serve you well!

If you're interested in progressing on to the EXP endurance program, you've already built a lot of the groundwork with the drills and exercises and have the new challenge of adding distance and developing late-run strength and the ability to run hard well past what you might consider today as fatigue. (We'll help you redefine what your personal quitting point looks like.) The SXP program also lends itself to any of the other programs: Total-Body Fitness, Building Muscle or Developing Strength. Whatever your next goal is, we've got an FXT program for you!

FXT:EXP

Building Endurance for Long-Distance Performance

Welcome to FXT:EXP, the next progression after finishing FXT:SXP to develop deep, powerful, muscle endurance for enhanced athletic performance. This program won't not be a walk in the park for anyone, whether they're incredibly fit amateurs or elite professional athletes. How can we say that? Quite simply, the tenacity you put into the program in the form of intensity from start to finish is up to each athlete.

If you're not totally smoked halfway through the program and fighting to keep your form (and maybe even keep your lunch down), then you aren't pushing yourself through what you consider "exhaustion" now. We added the quotes to reinforce that what you may consider exhaustion now—even after completing the difficult FXT:SXP program—is actually the period where you'll make most of your endurance gains.

There's a big attraction for many athletes to run a marathon, finish an Ironman Triathlon or even tackle an ultramarathon of 50 or even 100 (or more!) miles. While each of those events requires endurance, they're really at the more extreme end of the spectrum. A friendly tennis match, pick-up basketball game or soccer game requires a great deal of endurance. Heck, even maintaining your strength and focus during a round of golf can be taxing on most everyday athletes or weekend warriors. Using full-body training and, yes, running, we'll develop the strength and stamina to run or play better for even longer than you may have thought possible.

FXT:EXP is an intense regimen with elements from the FXT:FIT complete-body program along with many high-tempo plyometric moves and drills from the SXP speed performance program, all with timing and specificity to develop your athletic endurance. Prior to starting your timer and performing the first movement, commit yourself to completing the entire workout. Don't cheat your success by quitting early. Rest as needed and focus on your form—only stop when you can no longer perform each exercise properly or can no longer continue due to extreme fatigue, light-headedness, acute pain or other injury warning signs.

Completing FXT:SXP is a prerequisite for starting the FXT:EXP program because you'll be using more extreme versions of similar workouts you learned and mastered in FXT:SXP. Your mantra throughout this entire program should be: "Endurance is one of the most difficult disciplines, but it is the one who endures that the final victory comes" (Dean Karnazes).

You need to perform all the exercises to develop optimum performance endurance through functional fitness—don't skip exercises because you don't like them or they're difficult to complete. They were specifically chosen for their effectiveness at delivering results. In addition, finish every rep and set. Whether you're on pace to finish below the target time or double that amount, the only way you'll transform your mind and body is to develop consistency and tenacity from one workout to the next.

Developing endurance (and speed and total-body fitness, etc.) requires performing some exercises and drills at high intensity, but not all of them. You can't push your body 100% all the time, so follow the routine, including tempo and pace, and observe the proper rest periods.

Workouts That Develop Endurance

So, how do you train for endurance? Is it all long, slow running and repetition after repetition? Actually, no. We'll develop your endurance using some longer-distance running (or swimming, biking, hiking, jumping rope or whatever you choose as your cardio base-building) but we'll also use some performance-building techniques that will require proper form after what you may consider your point of exhaustion. Simply put, you'll be performing the hardest part of the workouts after you've already depleted your muscles of free glycogen and are running on fumes. Your goal is to finish the workouts even when you feel like giving up and re-establish your baseline for endurance and performance. Please note: This program will most likely be a lot different from what you may expect from an "endurance" type of regimen. Wrap your mind around the fact that we're looking at endurance like a 12-round MMA bout versus a 24-hour ultramarathon.

The exercises, drills and types of workouts you'll be using won't be all that different from SXP or FIT, but the application and timing for the most part will be specific to building endurance. Tempo runs will be longer, pick-up runs will be more intense and the ladders, reverse ladders and elevator workouts will challenge you mentally and physically to get to the very last rep.

See the "FXT:EXP Points Key" on page 106 to get a better understanding of how to calculate your FXT Score for each workout.

DEPLETION WORKOUTS: RUNNING ON EMPTY

Depletion runs are a rather extreme way that marathoners and triathletes develop endurance. They bring their bodies ever so close to failure, or "bonking" (when you run out of energy), and continue to push through the drills or exercises to complete the workout. Quite simply, these are workouts performed at high intensity and consistently completed with extraordinary maximum exertion—with no nutritional support. "Digging deep" barely describes the extreme nature of finishing a depletion workout when your body's glycogen is completely tapped out.

Depletion workouts are extreme and are only offered as an alternative program for

> **FXT:EXP TIP**—Finish at 110%. You'll get the most endurance-developing benefit out of the relatively short runs in this program by finishing the last 5–10 minutes near maximal effort. Even when your brain is sending signals of fatigue, your body still has the strength to finish strong, and even kick your final few minutes at an increased pace/harder intensity.

advanced athletes seeking to develop late-game or long-distance endurance when their energy reserves are nearly tapped. Professional athletes call this "the hurt locker" as this is the zone where races or games are ultimately decided. Elite athletes can "embrace the suck" longer and more proficiently than amateurs; this is one of the reasons they're on the podiums and winning championships, bringing home the MVP trophies.

To perform these workouts, you'll utilize a nutritional restriction called intermittent fasting. Essentially, you'll fast for about 12–16 hours before performing your workout, and then refuel immediately afterward. Optimally, these workouts should be performed as your last workout for the week (on Fridays), when you're planning to take both Saturday and Sunday off from training.

Note: Depletion workouts should be performed a maximum of once per week—stop exercising immediately if you become light-headed, delirious or experience any vertigo. These workouts should be performed with the guidance of a trainer or workout partner who is NOT performing them at the same time, paying close attention to the depleted athlete for any signs of erratic behavior. Always have a source of fast-burning carbs like an energy gel or candy bar on hand to refuel an athlete who's complaining of nausea or extreme light-headedness.

Nutrition for Building Endurance for Long-Distance Performance

Nutritional needs for endurance athletes are not necessarily different than those following the FXT:FIT or FXT:SXP programs (see FXT:FIT nutrition on page 174). The big difference is making sure you have enough slow-burning carbs in your diet to fuel you during longer workouts than you have most likely ever performed before. Unfortunately, there's no magic formula for what every athlete needs for sustained energy, and you'll need to do a little self-evaluation as you progress through the program. If you're really lethargic in the middle of a workout, you most likely are low on free glucose in your system and should add more

We refer to slow-burning carbs as brown or green carbs as a quick shortcut based on the predominant color of the carb source: brown carbs include sweet potato, whole grains and brown rice while green carbs cover all veggies. Fast-burning carbs are referred to as white carbs—simple, fast-burning sugar sources, like white bread, white rice, potatoes and even sugary energy gels, gummy bears or hard candy.

brown or green carbs about an hour before your workout. If you find yourself feeling bloated in the belly during a workout, you may be consuming too much, too near your workout.

After your FXT:EXP workout, you absolutely, positively need to refresh your fuel stores and begin muscle repair by eating or drinking a 4:1 ratio of fast-acting, white carbs and protein. Taking in simple sugars helps shuttle protein to your muscles to begin recovery and repair.

FXT:EXP POINTS KEY

20 Bodyweight Reps	=	5 FXT points
10 Weighted Reps	=	5 FXT points
Walk/Jog	=	3 FXT points/min
Moderate Run	=	5 FXT points/min
Hard Run/Sprint	=	7 FXT points/min

Ladders, Pyramids, sequential drills	=	5 FXT points /10 Reps
Hot Circuit 2	=	50 FXT points/round
Revolutions	=	50 FXT points/round
40s Drill	=	20 FXT points/round

Add up all your points to get your FXT Score.

INTENSITY:

If you finish above or below the Target Time, append the amount of time that you exceed over the Target Time to the end of your score.

Example: 20:00 Target Time, 22:00 finish = +2:00

EXAMPLE:

Basic Target Points: 80, Target Time: 16:00

Advanced Target Points: 120, Target Time: 18:00

Instructions: Complete as many sets as possible with good form. Rest as needed.

20 Bodyweight Squats = 5 points

1:00 Plank = 5 points

20 Lunges = 5 points

(20) Push-Ups = 5 points

Example: Completed 4 sets of the above in 20:00.

Score: 80 +4:00

FXT:EXP Program | Week 1

Warm up for 5 minutes prior to each workout; stretch after completion. Warm-Ups & Stretches start on page 166. Use exertion scale on page 67 for Easy, Moderate and Hard effort. Complete as many reps as possible with good form to reach Target Points & Target Time.

DAY 1

TARGET POINTS *Basic:* 90   *Advanced:* 120
TARGET TIME   *Basic:* 30:00   *Advanced:* 32:00

Exercise	Reps / Pts	Rounds	Time	Pts Total
1-Mile Run				

Basic: Easy Run, repeat 3x
Advanced: Moderate Run, repeat 4x

DAY 2

TARGET POINTS *Basic:* 60   *Advanced:* 120
TARGET TIME   *Basic:* 18:00   *Advanced:* 28:00

Exercise	Reps / Pts	Rounds	Time	Pts Total
Jumping Jacks *p. 142*	20 / 5			
Lunge *p. 150*	20 / 5			
T Push-Up *p. 140*	10 per side / 5			
Mountain Climber *p. 144*	20 / 5			
Thruster *p. 146*	10 / 5			
Box Jump *p. 155*	20 / 5			

Basic: 2x; *Advanced:* 4x

DAY 3

TARGET POINTS *Basic:* 120   *Advanced:* 150
TARGET TIME   *Basic:* 32:00   *Advanced:* 34:00

Exercise	Reps / Pts	Rounds	Time	Pts Total
1-Mile Run				
Jump Lunge *p. 150*	20 / 5			
Strider *p. 91*	10 per side / 5			

Basic: Easy Run, repeat 3x
Advanced: Moderate Run, repeat 4x

DAY 4

TARGET POINTS *Basic:* 60   *Advanced:* 100
TARGET TIME   *Basic:* 22:00   *Advanced:* 24:00

Exercise	Reps / Pts	Rounds	Time	Pts Total
Mason Twist *p. 133*	20 / 5			
Hip Raise *p. 141*	20 / 5			
Superman *p. 131*	20 / 5			
Plank *p. 136*	1:00 / 5			

Basic: 3x; *Advanced:* 5x

DAY 5

TARGET POINTS *Basic:* 60   *Advanced:* 90
TARGET TIME   *Basic:* 20:00   *Advanced:* 24:00

Exercise	Reps / Pts	Rounds	Time	Pts Total
1-Mile Run				

Basic: Easy Run, repeat 2x
Advanced: Moderate Run, repeat 3x

DAY 6

Rest

DAY 7

TARGET POINTS *Basic:* 105   *Advanced:* 175
TARGET TIME   *Basic:* 35:00   *Advanced:* 35:00

Exercise	Reps / Pts	Rounds	Time	Pts Total
35:00 Jog/Run				

Basic: Easy Run; *Advanced:* Moderate Run

FXT:EXP Program | Week 2

Warm up for 5 minutes prior to each workout; stretch after completion. Warm-Ups & Stretches start on page 166. Use exertion scale on page 67 for Easy, Moderate and Hard effort. Complete as many reps as possible with good form to reach Target Points & Target Time.

DAY 1

TARGET POINTS *Basic:* 90   *Advanced:* 120
TARGET TIME   *Basic:* 30:00   *Advanced:* 32:00

Exercise	Reps / Pts	Rounds	Time	Pts Total
1-Mile Run				

Basic: Easy Run, repeat 3x
Advanced: Moderate Run, repeat 4x

DAY 2

TARGET POINTS *Basic:* 60   *Advanced:* 120
TARGET TIME   *Basic:* 22:00   *Advanced:* 28:00

Exercise	Reps / Pts	Rounds	Time	Pts Total
Marching Twist p. 142	20 / 5			
Squat p. 148	20 / 5			
Wood Chop p. 134	20 / 5			
Inchworm p. 137	10 / 2.5			
Push-Up p. 156	10 / 2.5			
Box Jump p. 155	20 / 5			
Burpee p. 144	20 / 5			

Basic: 2x; *Advanced:* 4x

DAY 3

TARGET POINTS *Basic:* 100   *Advanced:* 150
TARGET TIME   *Basic:* 38:00   *Advanced:* 42:00

Exercise	Reps / Pts	Rounds	Time	Pts Total
Hot Circuit 2 p. 81	1/50			

Basic: 2x; *Advanced:* 3x

DAY 4

TARGET POINTS *Basic:* 60   *Advanced:* 100
TARGET TIME   *Basic:* 22:00   *Advanced:* 24:00

Exercise	Reps / Pts	Rounds	Time	Pts Total
Side Plank p. 137	:30 per side / 5			
Hip Raise p. 141	20 / 5			
In & Out p. 131	20 / 5			
Flutter Kick p. 134	20 / 5			

Basic: 3x; *Advanced:* 5x

DAY 5

TARGET POINTS *Basic:* 60   *Advanced:* 90
TARGET TIME   *Basic:* 20:00   *Advanced:* 24:00

Exercise	Reps / Pts	Rounds	Time	Pts Total
1-Mile Run				

Note: May be used as a "Depletion Run"

Basic: Easy Run, repeat 2x
Advanced: Moderate Run, repeat 3x

DAY 6

Rest

DAY 7

TARGET POINTS *Basic:* 105   *Advanced:* 175
TARGET TIME   *Basic:* 35:00   *Advanced:* 35:00

Exercise	Reps / Pts	Rounds	Time	Pts Total
35:00 Jog/Run				

Basic: Easy Run; *Advanced:* Moderate Run

Note: Basic Target Point assumes 3 points/min for easy run/walk 35:00, Adv. Target Point assumes 5 points/min for moderate run.

FXT:EXP Program | Week 3

Warm up for 5 minutes prior to each workout; stretch after completion. Warm-Ups & Stretches start on page 166. Use exertion scale on page 67 for Easy, Moderate and Hard effort. Complete as many reps as possible with good form to reach Target Points & Target Time.

DAY 1

TARGET POINTS *Basic:* 90   *Advanced:* 120
TARGET TIME   *Basic:* 30:00 *Advanced:* 32:00

Exercise	Reps / Pts	Rounds	Time	Pts Total
1-Mile Run				

Basic: Easy Run, repeat 3x
Advanced: Moderate Run, repeat 4x

DAY 2

TARGET POINTS *Basic:* 80   *Advanced:* 120
TARGET TIME   *Basic:* 28:00 *Advanced:* 32:00

Exercise	Reps / Pts	Rounds	Time	Pts Total
Box Jump *p. 155*	20 / 5			
Lunge *p. 150*	20 / 5			
Mountain Climber *p. 144*	20 / 5			
Mason Twist *p. 133*	20 / 5			
Side Plank *p. 137*	:30 per side / 5			
Superman *p. 131*	20 / 5			
Bicycle Crunch *p. 138*	20 / 5			
Thruster *p. 146*	10 / 5			

Basic: 2x; *Advanced:* 3x

DAY 3

TARGET POINTS *Basic:* 80   *Advanced:* 160
TARGET TIME   *Basic:* 35:00 *Advanced:* 48:00

Exercise	Reps / Pts	Rounds	Time	Pts Total
20/20 Drill *p. 91*	1 / 20			

Basic: 4x; *Advanced:* 8x

DAY 4

TARGET POINTS *Basic:* 140   *Advanced:* 170
TARGET TIME   *Basic:* 40:00 *Advanced:* 42:00

Exercise	Reps / Pts	Rounds	Time	Pts Total
10:00 Jump Rope *p. 165* Basic Skier Bell	1 / 50			
1-Mile Run				

Basic: Easy Run, repeat 3x
Advanced: Moderate Run, repeat 4x

DAY 5

TARGET POINTS *Basic:* 60   *Advanced:* 120
TARGET TIME   *Basic:* 20:00 *Advanced:* 32:00

Exercise	Reps / Pts	Rounds	Time	Pts Total
40s Drill *p. 81*	1 / 20			
1-Mile Run				

Basic: Easy Run, repeat 3x
Advanced: Moderate Run, repeat 4x

DAY 6

Rest

DAY 7

TARGET POINTS *Basic:* 135   *Advanced:* 225
TARGET TIME   *Basic:* 45:00 *Advanced:* 45:00

Exercise	Reps / Pts	Rounds	Time	Pts Total
45:00 Jog/Run				

Basic: Easy Run; *Advanced:* Moderate Run

FXT:EXP Program | Week 4

Warm up for 5 minutes prior to each workout; stretch after completion. Warm-Ups & Stretches start on page 166. Use exertion scale on page 67 for Easy, Moderate and Hard effort. Complete as many reps as possible with good form to reach Target Points & Target Time.

DAY 1

TARGET POINTS *Basic:* 90   *Advanced:* 120
TARGET TIME   *Basic:* 30:00   *Advanced:* 32:00

Exercise	Reps / Pts	Rounds	Time	Pts Total
1-Mile Run				

Basic: Easy Run, repeat 3x
Advanced: Moderate Run, repeat 4x

DAY 2

TARGET POINTS *Basic:* 80   *Advanced:* 120
TARGET TIME   *Basic:* 38:00   *Advanced:* 42:00

Exercise	Reps / Pts	Rounds	Time	Pts Total
Burpee *p. 144*	20 / 5			
Bizarro Burpee *p. 145*	20 / 5			
Bird Dog *p. 137*	10 / 2.5			
Hip Raise *p. 141*	10 / 2.5			
Box Jump *p. 155*	20 / 5			

Basic: 4x; *Advanced:* 6x

DAY 3

TARGET POINTS *Basic:* 50   *Advanced:* 100
TARGET TIME   *Basic:* 20:00   *Advanced:* 38:00

Exercise	Reps / Pts	Rounds	Time	Pts Total
Hill repeats: :20 Moderate Intensity :30 Walk/Rest :20 Hard Intensity :30 Walk/Rest	1 / 10			

Basic: 5x; *Advanced:* 10x

DAY 4

TARGET POINTS *Basic:* 105   *Advanced:* 140
TARGET TIME   *Basic:* 33:00   *Advanced:* 32:00

Exercise	Reps / Pts	Rounds	Time	Pts Total
Linear Reactive Step-Up *p. 154*	10 per side / 5			
Lunge *p. 150*	20 / 5			
Mountain Climber *p. 144*	20 / 5			
Mason Twist *p. 133*	20 / 5			
Side Plank *p. 137*	:30 per side / 5			
Superman *p. 131*	20 / 5			
Bicycle Crunch *p. 138*	20 / 5			

Basic: 3x; *Advanced:* 4x

DAY 5

TARGET POINTS *Basic:* 90   *Advanced:* 120
TARGET TIME   *Basic:* 30:00   *Advanced:* 32:00

Exercise	Reps / Pts	Rounds	Time	Pts Total
1-Mile Run				

Note: May be used as a "Depletion Run"

Basic: Easy Run, repeat 3x
Advanced: Tempo Run, repeat 4x

DAY 6

Rest

DAY 7

TARGET POINTS *Basic:* 135   *Advanced:* 225
TARGET TIME   *Basic:* 45:00   *Advanced:* 45:00

Exercise	Reps / Pts	Rounds	Time	Pts Total
45:00 Jog/Run				

Basic: Easy Run; *Advanced:* Moderate Run

FXT:EXP Program | Week 5

Warm up for 5 minutes prior to each workout; stretch after completion. Warm-Ups & Stretches start on page 166. Use exertion scale on page 67 for Easy, Moderate and Hard effort. Complete as many reps as possible with good form to reach Target Points & Target Time.

DAY 1

TARGET POINTS *Basic:* 90   *Advanced:* 120
TARGET TIME   *Basic:* 40:00   *Advanced:* 40:00

Exercise	Reps / Pts	Rounds	Time	Pts Total
1-Mile Run				

Basic: Easy Run, repeat 4x
Advanced: Moderate Run, repeat 5x

DAY 2

TARGET POINTS *Basic:* 90   *Advanced:* 180
TARGET TIME   *Basic:* 22:00   *Advanced:* 32:00

Exercise	Reps / Pts	Rounds	Time	Pts Total
Pyramid Seesaw: **1A** = Pyramid; **1B** = Reverse Pyramid				
1A: Landmine p. 163	1-5-1 / 15			
1B: Overhead Press p. 157	5-1-5 / 15			
1A: Deadlift p. 152	1-5-1 / 15			

Basic: 2x; *Advanced:* 4x

DAY 3

TARGET POINTS *Basic:* 80   *Advanced:* 160
TARGET TIME   *Basic:* 36:00   *Advanced:* 48:00

Exercise	Reps / Pts	Rounds	Time	Pts Total
20/20 Drill p. 91	1 / 20			

Basic: 4x; *Advanced:* 8x

DAY 4

TARGET POINTS *Basic:* 70   *Advanced:* 105
TARGET TIME   *Basic:* 22:00   *Advanced:* 24:00

Exercise	Reps / Pts	Rounds	Time	Pts Total
Box Jump p. 155	20 / 5			
Superman p. 131	20 / 5			
Mountain Climber p. 144	20 / 5			
Mason Twist p. 133	20 / 5			
Side Plank p. 137	:30 per side/5			
Jump Lunge p. 150	20 / 5			
Bicycle Crunch p. 138	20 / 5			

Basic: 2x; *Advanced:* 3x

DAY 5

TARGET POINTS *Basic:* 90   *Advanced:* 120
TARGET TIME   *Basic:* 30:00   *Advanced:* 32:00

Exercise	Reps / Pts	Rounds	Time	Pts Total
1-Mile Run				

Basic: Easy Run, repeat 3x
Advanced: Pick-Up Run, repeat 4x

DAY 6

Rest

DAY 7

TARGET POINTS *Basic:* 180   *Advanced:* 300
TARGET TIME   *Basic:* 60:00   *Advanced:* 60:00

Exercise	Reps / Pts	Rounds	Time	Pts Total
60:00 Jog/Run				

Basic: Easy Run; *Advanced:* Moderate Run

FXT:EXP Program | Week 6

Warm up for 5 minutes prior to each workout; stretch after completion. Warm-Ups & Stretches start on page 166. Use exertion scale on page 67 for Easy, Moderate and Hard effort. Complete as many reps as possible with good form to reach Target Points & Target Time.

DAY 1

TARGET POINTS *Basic:* 90   *Advanced:* 120
TARGET TIME   *Basic:* 40:00   *Advanced:* 40:00

Exercise	Reps / Pts	Rounds	Time	Pts Total
1-Mile Run				

Basic: Easy Run, repeat 4x
Advanced: Moderate Run, repeat 5x

DAY 2

TARGET POINTS *Basic:* 120   *Advanced:* 240
TARGET TIME   *Basic:* 22:00   *Advanced:* 32:00

Exercise	Reps / Pts	Rounds	Time	Pts Total
Pyramid Seesaw: **1A** = Pyramid; **1B** = Reverse Pyramid				
Pyramid Seesaw	1 / 45			
1B: Lunge with Biceps Curl p. 151	5-1-5 / 15			
1B: Ball Thruster p. 147	5-1-5 / 15			
1A: Push-Up p. 156	1-5-1 / 15			
1A: In & Out p. 131	1-5-1 / 15			

Basic: 2x; *Advanced:* 4x

DAY 3

TARGET POINTS *Basic:* 135   *Advanced:* 150
TARGET TIME   *Basic:* 27:00   *Advanced:* 21:00

Exercise	Reps / Pts	Rounds	Time	Pts Total
1-Mile Run	1 / 20			

Basic: Moderate Run, repeat 3x
Advanced: Hard Run, repeat 3x

DAY 4

TARGET POINTS *Basic:* 60   *Advanced:* 80
TARGET TIME   *Basic:* 24:00   *Advanced:* 32:00

Exercise	Reps / Pts	Rounds	Time	Pts Total
Burpee p. 144	20 / 5			
Bizarro Burpee p. 145	20 / 5			
Bird Dog p. 137	10 / 2.5			
Hip Raise p. 141	10 / 2.5			
Box Jump p. 155	20 / 5			

Basic: 3x; *Advanced:* 4x

DAY 5

TARGET POINTS *Basic:* 90   *Advanced:* 120
TARGET TIME   *Basic:* 30:00   *Advanced:* 32:00

Exercise	Reps / Pts	Rounds	Time	Pts Total
1-Mile Run				

Note: May be used as a "Depletion Run"

Basic: Easy Run, repeat 3x
Advanced: Tempo Run, repeat 4x

DAY 6

Rest

DAY 7

TARGET POINTS *Basic:* 180   *Advanced:* 300
TARGET TIME   *Basic:* 60:00   *Advanced:* 60:00

Exercise	Reps / Pts	Rounds	Time	Pts Total
60:00 Jog/Run				

Basic: Easy Run; *Advanced:* Moderate Run

FXT:EXP Program | Week 7

Warm up for 5 minutes prior to each workout; stretch after completion. Warm-Ups & Stretches start on page 166. Use exertion scale on page 67 for Easy, Moderate and Hard effort. Complete as many reps as possible with good form to reach Target Points & Target Time.

DAY 1

TARGET POINTS *Basic:* 90   *Advanced:* 120
TARGET TIME   *Basic:* 40:00   *Advanced:* 40:00

Exercise	Reps / Pts	Rounds	Time	Pts Total
1-Mile Run				

Basic: Easy Run, repeat 4x
Advanced: Moderate Run, repeat 5x

DAY 2

TARGET POINTS *Basic:* 100   *Advanced:* 150
TARGET TIME   *Basic:* 30:00   *Advanced:* 42:00

Exercise	Reps / Pts	Rounds	Time	Pts Total
Hot Circuit 2 *p. 81*	1 / 50			

Basic: 2x; *Advanced:* 3x

DAY 3

TARGET POINTS *Basic:* 80   *Advanced:* 160
TARGET TIME   *Basic:* 36:00   *Advanced:* 48:00

Exercise	Reps / Pts	Rounds	Time	Pts Total
20/20 Drill *p. 91*	1 / 20			

Basic: 4x; *Advanced:* 8x

DAY 4

TARGET POINTS *Basic:* 45   *Advanced:* 60
TARGET TIME   *Basic:* 32:00   *Advanced:* 36:00

Exercise	Reps / Pts	Rounds	Time	Pts Total
Ladder Seesaw: **1A** = Ladder; **1B** = Reverse Ladder				
1A: Roll-Out *p. 136*	1-5 / 7.5			
1B: Pull-Up *p. 156*	5-1 / 7.5			

Basic: 3x; *Advanced:* 4x

DAY 5

TARGET POINTS *Basic:* 130   *Advanced:* 180
TARGET TIME   *Basic:* 40:00   *Advanced:* 46:00

Exercise	Reps / Pts	Rounds	Time	Pts Total
1-Mile Run				
1:00 Rest				
Push-Up *p. 156*	20 / 5			
Hip Raise *p. 141*	20 / 5			
Jump Lunge *p. 150*	20 / 5			
Flutter Kick *p. 134*	20 / 5			

Basic: 2x; *Advanced:* 3x

DAY 6

Rest

DAY 7

TARGET POINTS *Basic:* 270   *Advanced:* 450
TARGET   *Basic:* 90:00   *Advanced:* 90:00

Exercise	Reps / Pts	Rounds	Time	Pts Total
90:00 Jog/Run				

Basic: Easy Run; *Advanced:* Moderate Run

FXT:EXP Program | Week 8

Warm up for 5 minutes prior to each workout; stretch after completion. Warm-Ups & Stretches start on page 166. Use exertion scale on page 67 for Easy, Moderate and Hard effort. Complete as many reps as possible with good form to reach Target Points & Target Time.

DAY 1

TARGET POINTS *Basic:* 90   *Advanced:* 120
TARGET   *Basic:* 40:00   *Advanced:* 40:00

Exercise	Reps / Pts	Rounds	Time	Pts Total
1-Mile Run				

Note: May be used as a "Depletion Run"

Basic: Easy Run, repeat 4x
Advanced: Moderate Run, repeat 5x

DAY 2

TARGET POINTS *Basic:* 80   *Advanced:* 120
TARGET TIME   *Basic:* 20:00   *Advanced:* 32:00

Exercise	Reps / Pts	Rounds	Time	Pts Total
40s Drill *p. 81*	1 / 20			

Basic: 4x; *Advanced:* 6x

DAY 3

TARGET POINTS *Basic:* 50   *Advanced:* 100
TARGET TIME   *Basic:* 20:00   *Advanced:* 38:00

Exercise	Reps / Pts	Rounds	Time	Pts Total

Hill repeats:
  :20 Moderate
    Intensity
  :30 Walk/Rest
  :20 Hard Intensity
  :30 Walk/Rest
	1 / 10			

Basic: 5x; *Advanced:* 10x

DAY 4

TARGET POINTS *Basic:* 120   *Advanced:* 240
TARGET TIME   *Basic:* 16:00   *Advanced:* 22:00

Exercise	Reps / Pts	Rounds	Time	Pts Total
Pyramid Seesaw: **1A** = Pyramid; **1B** = Reverse Pyramid				
1A: V-Sit *p. 132*	5-1-5 / 15			
1A: Ball Thruster *p. 147*	1-5-1 / 15			
1B: Push-Up *p. 156*	5-1-5 / 15			
1B: In & Out *p. 131*	1-5-1 / 15			

Basic: 2x; *Advanced:* 3x

DAY 5

TARGET POINTS *Basic:* 110   *Advanced:* 170
TARGET TIME   *Basic:* 35:00   *Advanced:* 28:00

Exercise	Reps / Pts	Rounds	Time	Pts Total
3-Mile Run				
1:00 Rest				
Plank *p. 136*	1:00 / 5			
Hip Raise *p. 141*	20 / 5			
In & Out *p. 131*	20 / 5			
Box Jump *p. 155*	20 / 5			

Basic: 2x; *Advanced:* 3x

DAY 6

Rest

DAY 7

TARGET POINTS *Basic:* 270   *Advanced:* 450
TARGET TIME   *Basic:* 90:00   *Advanced:* 90:00

Exercise	Reps / Pts	Rounds	Time	Pts Total
90:00 Jog/Run				

Basic: Easy Run; *Advanced:* Moderate Run

Success!

Congratulations on finishing the FXT:EXP endurance performance program! We're sure you now realize this was more intense than you'd expect from an "endurance" program, right? By completing the workouts and drills, you've taken your athletic performance to a place where you can compete at a higher level for much longer than ever before. The full-body strength that you've developed through completing this program can be applied to any physical activity, from pick-up hoops to 18 (or 36) holes on the links. It may even improve your free throws or driving distance. Of course, your sport-specific skill level has a lot to do with how you perform, but increased total-body conditioning will help you jump, run or swing a club longer, and a strong, flexible core means more power.

So, what's next? Once you've completed any program in this book, it's a perfect time to reflect on your progress and re-evaluate your goals. If you don't feel like you performed up to your full potential or want to progress even farther on a particular regimen, then by all means do it again. Our recommendation is to not do any one particular program more than twice back to back, as this may lead to overuse injuries, plateaus or mental burn-out. The programs in this book were all crafted together to provide a year-round series of workouts to develop periods of muscle and strength growth, and total-body conditioning through calisthenics, speed drills and endurance training. Pick a program, commit to it, and keep progressing to develop a whole new you!

FXT:MX1
Building Muscle

"Look better naked." There are very few things in life that don't benefit from ruthless simplification. When you're trying to state your goal, try to see if yours is about looking better naked. If so, you probably want to build muscle. Seriously, take some time and think about it.

Now that you're back and still reading, we're going to go over the simplest way known to man to build rock-solid muscle. There are literally thousands of approaches to muscle building—we've gone over most of them, distilled them down to their essence, taken the good, thrown away the bad and built a lifelong program to put on slabs of muscle.

But just because this is simple doesn't mean it's going to be easy. It won't be. You still need to put in the work and time, as well as follow the nutritional advice. If you do this and pay close attention to how you respond, you'll get results.

A special note to women: We've been asked in the past if this program is just for men. Absolutely not! Everything we talk about equally applies to women. The big difference is the time it will take as well as the expected results. Women often say they "don't want to get bulky" as a reason they typically don't lift weights. Now think about it this way: How many men WANT to look bulky but find it's difficult to actually do it? Ladies, there is near-zero chance you'll get bulky by lifting weights. Instead, you'll tighten up, build dense muscle and start to have a very athletic look. Don't worry about looking like a man—it's not going to happen.

How to Use the Program

Take a quick peek at the FXT:MX1 workout starting on page 121. Notice that the program is one week in length. We bet you're saying to yourself, "What the heck, guys? You told me all the programs were eight weeks long." Our answer is pretty simple: "Yes, they're eight weeks long. Just take a deep breath and read on."

FXT:MX1 is designed as a progressive routine to be performed by intermediate and advanced athletes five times a week over eight weeks, equaling 40 total workouts. All athletes, especially beginners, should take this program at their own pace, utilizing weights that they can easily perform all the required reps and progress steadily toward the five-days-per-week goal. Beginners are encouraged to take one day off between workouts for as many weeks as needed while keeping to the goal of 40 completed workouts before re-evaluating their workout regimen as outlined on page 36. Take the FXT:MX1 baseline test on page 61 to give you an idea of the target weights you should be using for each type of movement.

Repeat this five-day workout following the Basic or Advanced Target FXT Points for eight weeks, increasing your weights or reps by no more than 15% for a specific lift per week.

Training Styles That Build Muscle

The formula for building muscle (and by that we mean muscle size) is progressive resistance (strength training), sufficient volume (volume training) and muscular tension (tension training). You'll need to lift sufficient weights to tax your muscles, at a volume that promotes growth, for a certain amount of time to stress the muscle fibers. When you combine these factors together, you'll be creating an environment for muscle growth like no other.

Now let's look at these types of training separately. Each style has a base philosophy that can achieve decent results by itself, but combined they're even more effective. Understanding each style's strengths and weaknesses will allow you to understand when and where to use them effectively.

STRENGTH TRAINING

Classic strength training is only concerned with increasing the amount of weight a person can lift. In powerlifting this is achieved through body position, hand, foot and bar positions, as well as adding suits. We won't be doing any of that, though we will try to increase core strength.

STRENGTH: increasing base strength, fun program to follow, ego boosting

WEAKNESS: increasing muscle size

Strength has many advantages and should be the base of any good hypertrophy program. One of the failings of pure volume or tension programs is that they don't incorporate a strength component. And while volume and tension training can be more effective at increasing muscle size than strength training alone, combined they achieve more than they could apart.

Our approach to strength training is called progressive overloading, meaning we'll continually strive to add more weight to the bar for a prescribed set of reps and sets. In practice we want someone to add weight each workout as long as you can continue to hit your reps and sets number. When you can no longer lift for the prescribed reps in a set, you hold steady until you can. This means you'll be taxing your muscles each and every workout in a progressive way. You should be able to continually achieve new maximum lifts for quite some time using this approach. This method is naturally immune to stagnation as you'll theoretically never be doing the same workout twice. There is, of course, an upper limit on just how strong you

can get, although you need not worry—it will take quite some time before you find this ceiling. Bottom line: You'll always be trying to move up in weight for strength-training sets.

VOLUME TRAINING

Volume training is primarily concerned with the overall volume (meaning number of reps and sets) per workout. To achieve a higher number of reps and sets, the overall weight of exercises needs to be reduced, sometimes by as much as 50 to 70 percent, depending on the muscle group being worked. Volume training is where you'll feel the "pump" that you might hear others talk about. What happens is the muscles get a rush of blood from all the activity and grow accordingly. Of course, this "pump" is only temporary but the results of increasing the overall load on the muscle will be eventual growth.

STRENGTH: increasing muscle size, great for combination lifts

WEAKNESS: increasing muscle strength, needing to check your ego

An aspect of volume training that's often overlooked is the ego issue. You'll be lifting much lighter weights than your 1-rep or 5-rep max and you'll be using very strict form. You'll see others around the gym bouncing heavy weights and you'll be tempted to give in to your ego and start to increase the weights. However, this will be a huge mistake and will only hurt you in the long run. Be sure of yourself and the approach—be consistent and you'll achieve more than those people bouncing heavy weights. It's commonly said that when you bounce heavy weights, the only thing that grows is your ego.

Our approach to volume training is pretty classic. Volume training works well for most muscles but best for the big movers. Legs, chest and shoulders all respond well to volume training. Smaller muscles achieve good results through volume training but we have a better approach for them later. For now we'll keep the volume for the bigger muscle groups.

Finally, you won't move up in weight when volume training until you can do the prescribed number of reps and sets. That's the nature of volume training: The reps and sets are more important than the weight.

TENSION TRAINING

Classic tension training has two main components: time under tension and constant tension. Time under tension, or TUT, deals with the total time a muscle is worked, meaning total number of seconds in a work set. Constant tension means keeping tension on the muscle for the entire work set, meaning you won't lock out fully during a set.

> **STRENGTH:** increasing muscle size and hardness, particularly in isolation exercises

> **WEAKNESS:** extremely taxing on central nervous system, requires extreme mental fortitude

Tension-training programs typically incorporate either or both of these approaches. Our approach will blend them into one tension work set called Rest-Pause.

Rest-Pause is a tension style in which, for a certain lift, you keep constant tension on the muscle being worked for the entire work set—you never fully lock out and you use very slow and methodical movement. The movement should be 5 to 8 seconds down, 1 to 2 seconds up—no bouncing of the weights ever! This is how a rest-pause set will look:

1. You work the exercise to failure, at which point you release tension by putting the weight down.

2. Now take 10–15 deep breaths and then start the exercise again for as many reps as you can, again putting the weight down when you reach failure.

3. Take another 10–15 deep breaths and go once more until failure.

That's considered one Rest-Pause set. The total number of reps you do between the pauses is the total number for the Rest-Pause set. In practice, a typical Rest-Pause set might be 8 reps, a 10-second pause, 4 reps, a 10-second pause, and 2 reps—for a total of 14 reps.

You progress in a Rest-Pause set by meeting certain rep requirements for a certain weight. We say that once you achieve 15 reps at a certain weight, feel free to move up in weight for the next workout. However, if you fail to get 10 reps at the new weight, go back down to the previous weight until you reach 18 or 20 reps. This is how you bust through plateaus in Rest-Pause exercises.

As with volume training, you'll be using much less weight than your 1-rep or 5-rep max. Resist the urge to cheat, bounce weight or decrease the time on the descent. This is the single most common mistake with both volume and tension training and it hurts overall progress in the long run.

Nutrition for Building Muscle

Nutrition plays a big part in fueling for training and getting the long-term body composition you want. Refer to "Nutrition for Building Muscle and Developing Strength" on page 176 for guidelines on meal timing and macro- and micronutrient consumption. You'll also learn how what you take in before, during and after training affects your success.

FXT:MX1 KEY TERMS

Warm-Up: Warm-up set

Normal: Normal body-building set

Drop Set: Single Drop set after previous set

Power: Explosive power, 1 second up, 2–3 second down

Rest-Pause: Single working set to failure, 5 deep breaths, go again. Do this 3 times.

AMAN: As Many as Needed

AMAP: As Many as Possible

FXT:MX1 POINTS KEY

10 Weighted Reps   = 5 FXT points

20 Bodyweight Reps = 5 FXT points

EXAMPLE:

Basic Target Points: 80, Target Time: 16:00

Advanced Target Points: 120, Target Time: 18:00

Instructions: Complete as many sets as possible with good form. Rest as needed.

20 Bodyweight Squats = 5 points

1:00 Plank = 5 points

20 Lunges = 5 points

(20) Push-Ups = 5 points

Example: Completed 4 sets of the above in 20:00.

Score: 80 +4:00

Note: FXT:MX1 does not have a Target Time, as the workout has required time under tension and is designed to be performed while focusing on form rather than completion time. See the chart on page 62 for guidelines on how much weight you should be targeting based on a percentage of your body weight.

FXT:MX1 Program | Weeks 1–8

DAY 1 Chest (Major), Shoulders (minor), Triceps (minor)

TARGET POINTS *Basic:* 75   *Advanced:* 140
TOTAL REPS *Basic:* 200   *Advanced:* 280

Exercise	Style	Sets	Reps	Alternate
Bench Press p. 162	Warm-Up	3	10–20	
Bench Press	Normal	5	5	
Bench Press	Volume	5	12–20	
Overhead Press p. 157	Volume	5	12–20	Lateral Raise
Dip p. 160	Normal	5	AMAP	

DAY 2 Back (Major), Quads (minor), Biceps (minor)

TARGET POINTS *Basic:* 75   *Advanced:* 105
TOTAL REPS *Basic:* 150   *Advanced:* 210

Exercise	Style	Sets	Reps	Alternate
Deadlift p. 152	Warm-Up	AMAN	5	
Deadlift	Reverse Pyramid	5	3, 3, 5, 5, 5	
Leg Press p. 164	Volume	3	15–20	Front Squat
Barbell Row p. 158	Normal	3	8	1-Arm DB Row
DB Shrug p. 159	Normal	3	8–10	
Barbell Curl p. 158	Normal	3	8–10	

DAY 3 Core, Glutes

TARGET POINTS *Basic:* 70   *Advanced:* 140
TOTAL SETS *Basic:* 2   *Advanced:* 4

Exercise	Style	Sets	Reps	Points/Set
Hip Raise p. 141	Normal		20	10
Bird Dog p. 137	Normal		20	5
Plank p. 136	Normal		5	5
Landmine p. 163	Normal		20	10
Wood Chop p. 134	Normal		20	5

DAY 4 Shoulders (major), Chest (minor), Triceps (Minor)

TARGET POINTS *Basic:* 90   *Advanced:* 110
TOTAL SETS *Basic:* 180   *Advanced:* 220

Exercise	Style	Sets	Reps	Alternate
Overhead Press p. 157	Warm-Up	3	10	
Overhead Press	Normal	3	5	
Overhead Press	Volume	5	15–20	
Bench Press p. 162	Normal	3	8–12	Incline Bench Press
Triceps Pressdown p. 164	Normal	3	8–10	Triceps Kickback
Shoulder Raise p. 161	Rest–Pause	1	12–15	

DAY 5 Legs (Major)

TARGET POINTS *Basic:* 115   *Advanced:* 170
TOTAL SETS *Basic:* 230   *Advanced:* 340

Exercise	Style	Sets	Reps	Alternate
Squat p. 148	Warm-Up	3	12–15	
Squat p. 148	Warm-Up	3	10–15	
Squat p. 148	Warm-Up	AMAN	5	Front Squat
Squat p. 148	Reverse Pyramid	5	3, 3, 5, 5, 5	Front Squat
Leg Press p. 164	Volume	3	12–20	Squat
Romanian Deadlift p. 153	Normal	3	8–12	
Hamstring Curl p. 164	Normal	5	8–12	
Calf Raise p. 154	Normal	3	15–20	

DAYS 6 & 7

Rest

Success!

Awesome! You've gotten through the FXT:MX1 program and are well on your way to building solid, lifelong quality muscle. Remember to keep the long view and not get discouraged by any small stalls or missteps along the way. Building muscle is hard, but you now have the information needed to develop the body you've always wanted.

FXT:ST1
Developing Strength

"I want to look better naked" is a great way to decipher whether or not your goal is to put on muscle. It's a bit trickier to simplify a strength goal. Sometimes the goal is "I want to get better at my sport," or "I want to dunk a basketball," or perhaps "I want to increase my bench press/squat/deadlift." They all really boil down to strength. Think about your goal and put it through those filters. If all else fails, pit "look better naked" against your stated goal. If "look better naked" doesn't win outright, you likely want to build strength.

Now that we've established that you indeed want to build strength, how do you do it? The good news is developing strength is much more straightforward than building muscle, where there are many more variables at play. Strength is much more linear and can be distilled down to simpler principles. The program we've outlined incorporates fewer variations compared to our muscle-building program (page 116) and more base principles to build a simple yet effective program. However, make no mistake—you'll still need to work hard. Developing strength is about lifting weights near the upper limit of your current strength to push that upper limit higher and higher. That can be uncomfortable, but you'll need to stick with it to get stronger.

Note that strength can come in waves. Someone new to lifting will likely see dramatic improvement very quickly, plateau, break through the plateau and then see more improvement at a diminished rate to the initial strength gains. A seasoned lifter will likely see slower strength gains to the novice lifter and this can be discouraging. So you'll need mental strength as well. You'll need to look at the big picture, set some goals and work toward them. Keep on marching toward your goal and keep learning about your body in the process. Trust us—you'll hit your goals and it will all be worth it.

How to Use the Program

Take a quick peek at the FXT:ST1 workout starting on page 128. Notice that the program is one week in length. We bet you're saying to yourself, "What the heck, guys? You told me all the programs were eight weeks long." Our

ESTIMATING YOUR 1RM

There's no perfect way to calculate your 1RM without actually testing your 1RM (via a lift), though we can estimate it using a simple formula.

To estimate your 1RM, take the weight in pounds

x .0333

x reps

+ weight.

EXAMPLE: A 225-pound back squat for 10 reps would estimate your 1RM at 300 pounds.

225lbs

x .0333

x 10 reps

+ 225lbs

= estimated 1RM of 300lbs

answer is pretty simple: "Yes, they're eight weeks long. Just take a deep breath and read on."

FXT:ST1 is designed as a progressive routine to be performed by intermediate and advanced athletes five times a week over eight weeks, equaling 40 total workouts. All athletes, especially beginners, should take this program at their own pace, utilizing weights that they can easily perform all the required reps and progress steadily toward the five-days-per-week goal. Beginners are encouraged to take one day off between workouts for as many weeks as needed while keeping to the goal of 40 completed workouts before re-evaluating their workout regimen as outlined on page 36. Take the FXT:ST1 baseline test on page 61 to get an idea of the target weights you should be using for each type of movement.

Repeat this five-day workout following the Basic or Advanced Target FXT Points for eight weeks, increasing your weights or reps by no more than 15% for a specific lift per week.

Rules for Developing Strength

We said that developing strength is pretty easy. The challenge comes in wading through all the information out there and actually building a program. There are many programs that talk about different sets, rep ranges and percentage of XRM (e.g., 1-, 3- or 5-rep max) and which is better. Unless you're trying to go from elite to pro, or near-Olympian to Olympian, it likely doesn't matter. Sounds a bit like heresy, right? It isn't. All the programs work. They really do.

If you have a preference, stop reading this and just go with the one you like the best. What we're going to prescribe is the strength-training style we feel is the best for the majority of people. That's not to say this program can't take you from elite to pro or near-Olympian to Olympian, because it can. However, at that level you'll have access to personalized nutrition and training programs that can work for you individually. There's just no substitute for personalized programming.

This program is simple with some very simple rules to follow. Once you nail down these rules, you can walk into the gym each and every day, ready to tackle the weights.

1. START LIGHT

You'll have much more long-term success with a solid foundation than a shaky one. A solid foundation is built by starting with less weight than you can really handle and making absolutely certain you're ready to rock and roll. We're serious—don't let your ego get in the way. Start light, nail your form, make sure you

STRATEGIES TO OVERCOME PLATEAUS AND STALLS

1. Smaller wins: Back the weight off by 2.5 pounds at the next workout. When you nail this, add 2.5 to the next workout (back to stalled weight).

2. Back the weight off 5 pounds for two workouts, use shorter rest periods and nail all 5 reps of all 5 sets.

3. Scale back the weight to 75% of your stalled weight and do 3–5 sets of 10 reps. This should still be very challenging, though in a different way.

4. 50% sets: Take the stalled weight to failure. Rest 60 seconds. Do another set, aiming to get half of the reps you performed before reaching failure ("failed reps"). Rest 60 seconds. Do a final set to failure, aiming to get 50% of the second set of failed reps. Keep going if you feel good. A sample 50% set might be bench press at 150 pounds for 6 reps, 3 reps, 2 reps (50% of 3 is 1.5, so go ahead and do 2!) and 1 rep.

5. In extreme stalls, switch the exercise for two workouts. For instance, change flat bench to incline bench (you'll need a different weight, of course).

know what you're doing and progressively work up to weights that are challenging.

Our recommendation is to start with 50% of your 1-rep max (1RM) for your first workout. This means that if you bench press 150 pounds for 1 rep, your first workout will be 75 pounds, which is a 45-pound Olympic bar with 15 pounds on each side. For each workout, add 5 pounds (2.5 pounds per side) to the bar.

Quite honestly, this is going to be an exercise in humility for most people, but it's worth it. In a few short workouts you'll have a very challenging workout, but you'll also have a base of good form, strength and confidence to annihilate this and all future workouts!

2. BASIC COMPOUND MOVEMENTS

We're going to focus on basic compound movements like the bench press, overhead press, squat and deadlift for the main lift of each workout, with some other exercises thrown in for accessory work. The rule should be that you focus on exercises that work more muscles and avoid those that isolate them. The one caveat would be on accessory work: Feel free to use an isolation exercise to bring up a lagging body part.

3. OVER-WARM-UP

We don't see this used very often in strength programs but we've found this to be very effective. For your warm-up, progress as you normally would, except warm up past your intended working sets for the last warm-up set. For example, if your working set for the day is the 225-pound bench press, your warm-up might look like this: bar x 20 reps, 135 x 12–15 reps, 185 x 8 reps, 225 x 5 reps, 250 x 2–3 reps. You then back off the weight to 225 for your work sets of 5x5.

4. PROGRESSIVE RESISTANCE

Each workout is going to be different. The basis of this program is a very simple 5x5 (5 sets of 5 reps) at its core. To make progress you need to move up weight each workout. The technical rule is you need to hit all 5 reps in all 5 sets to move up in weight.

At some point, you'll fail to hit all 5 sets of all 5 reps. Sorry, that's just the nature of the game. That means the next workout will be the same weight and you'll be shooting for all

---

FXT:ST1 KEY TERMS

Warm-Up: Warm-up set

Normal: Normal body-building set

AMAN: As Many as Needed

AMAP: As Many as Possible

Over-Warm-Up: Warm up over your working sets

FXT:ST1 POINTS KEY

10 Weighted Reps = 5 FXT points

20 Bodyweight Reps = 5 FXT points

EXAMPLE:

Basic Target Points: 80, Target Time: 16:00

Advanced Target Points: 120, Target Time: 18:00

Instructions: Complete as many sets as possible with good form. Rest as needed.

20 Bodyweight Squats = 5 points

1:00 Plank = 5 points

20 Lunges = 5 points

(20) Push-Ups = 5 points

Example: Completed 4 sets of the above in 20:00.

Score: 80 +4:00

Note: FXT:MX1 does not have a Target Time, as the workout has required time under tension and is designed to be performed while focusing on form rather than completion time. See the chart on page 62 for guidelines on how much weight you should be targeting based on a percentage of your body weight.

5 reps in all 5 sets again. You might hit it, you might not. Just don't move up until you hit all 5 reps of all 5 sets.

5. LOG EVERYTHING

Unless you're a human computer, you'll forget something. Keep a log book for your workouts and make sure you write everything down. We even recommend you write down how you felt in the workout. Did everything feel great? Write it down. Did you struggle on reps 4 and 5 of the last set of the overhead press? Write it down. Did you notice a dip in your left side compared to your right side? Write it down.

We HIGHLY recommend you use the FXT:FIT mobile app or log sheets to keep track of your progress and workout data.

6. ACCESSORIZE

Each workout should be about the main strength exercise of the day (i.e., deadlift, squat, overhead press or bench press). The rest of the workout should be about bringing up deficiencies. Are you weak off the ground in the deadlift? Work on exercises that help this. Are your glutes weak? Spend time on them. Pay attention to your body and what it's trying to tell you. When the weights start to get heavier, all the small details matter much more.

7. STICK WITH IT

Of course, the single most important rule: Stick with it. Keep going even when you plateau. Keep plugging along when the gains are slower. Keep pushing.

Nutrition for Developing Strength

Nutrition plays a big part in fueling for training and getting the long-term body composition you want. Refer to "Nutrition for Building Muscle and Developing Strength" on page 176 for guidelines on meal timing and macro- and micronutrient consumption. You'll also learn about how what you take in before, during and after training affects your success.

FXT:ST1 Program | Weeks 1–8

DAY 1 Chest (Major), Shoulders (minor), Triceps (minor)

TARGET POINTS *Basic:* 110   Advanced: 160
TOTAL REPS   *Basic:* 220   Advanced: 320

Exercise	Sets	Reps	Notes
Bench Press *p. 162* OR Incline Bench Press *p. 163*	AMAN	5	Over-warm-up
Bench Press *p. 162*	5	5	
Incline DB Bench Press *p. 163* OR Chest Fly *p. 161* OR Dip *p. 160*	5	12–20	Alternate "chest accessory" exercise each week
Overhead Press *p. 157* OR Lateral Shoulder Raise *p. 161* OR Front Shoulder Raise *p. 161*	5	12–20	Alternate "shoulder accessory" exercise each week
Dip *p. 160*	5	AMAP	Squeeze at top and lower slowly

DAY 2 Back (Major), Accessory

TARGET POINTS *Basic:* 90   Advanced: 120
TOTAL REPS   *Basic:* 180   Advanced: 240

Exercise	Sets	Reps	Notes
Deadlift *p. 152*	AMAN	5	Over-warm-up
Deadlift	5	5	
Romanian Deadlift *p. 153* OR Good Morning *p. 152*	3	10–15	Alternate "deficiency accessory" exercise each week
Barbell Row *p. 159* OR 1-Arm DB Row *p. 159*	3	10–15	
Chin-Up *p. 157* OR Pull-up *p. 156*	3	8–10	If 3 sets of 10 are easy, add a weight vest
Barbell Curl *p. 158*	3	15–25	Be sure to squeeze biceps at top of each rep, lower slowly

DAY 3 Core, Glutes

TARGET POINTS *Basic:* 90   Advanced: 150
TOTAL SETS   *Basic:* 3   Advanced: 5

Exercise	Sets	Reps	Points
Hip Raise *p. 141*		20	10
Good Morning *p. 152*		20	10
Plank *p. 136*		1:00	5
Swoop & Touch *p. 131*		20	5

DAY 4 Shoulders (major), Chest & Shoulder (accessory), Triceps (Minor)			
TARGET POINTS *Basic:* 100 Advanced: 200 TOTAL SETS *Basic:* 200 Advanced: 300			
Exercise	Sets	Reps	Notes
Overhead Press *p. 157*	AMAN	5	Over-warm-up
Overhead Press	5	5	
Incline Bench Press *p. 163* OR Chest Fly *p. 161* OR Dip *p. 160*	5	12–20	Alternate "chest accessory" exercise each week; use different exercise than Monday
Overhead Press *p. 157* OR Lateral Shoulder Raise *p. 161* OR Front Shoulder Raise *p. 161*	5	12–20	Alternate "shoulder accessory" exercise each week; use different exercise than Monday
Triceps Pressdown *p. 164* OR Triceps Kickback *p. 160*	3	failure	Use a light weight, target 15–25 reps
Shoulder Raise *p. 161*	1	failure	Use a light weight, shoot for 25 reps
DAY 5 Legs (Major)			
TARGET POINTS *Basic:* 130 Advanced: 165 TOTAL SETS *Basic:* 260 Advanced: 330			
Exercise	Sets	Reps	Notes
Squat *p. 148*	3	12–15	
Squat	3	10	
Squat OR Front Squat *p. 149*	AMAN	5	Over-warm-up
Squat	5	5	
Leg Press *p. 164*	4	8–15	Use one leg if possible; alternate each set
Romanian Deadlift *p. 153*	3	8–12	
Hamstring Curl *p. 164*	5	8–12	
Calf Raise *p. 154*	3	15–20	
DAYS 6 & 7			
Rest			

Success!

And you're done! That was simple, wasn't it? Joking, of course, but we do hope we've taken the mystery out of getting stronger. Along the way we've given some strategies to break through plateaus and propel you to strength levels you've never seen before. Congratulations! Keep your head up and weight moving. Before you know it you'll be throwing around numbers you previously only dreamed about.

PART 3: EXERCISES

Cobra

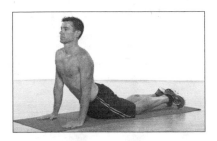

Lying on your stomach, place your hands directly under your shoulders with your fingers facing forward and straighten your legs and point your toes. Exhale and engage your core while lifting your chest off the floor and pushing your hips gently into the floor. Your arms help guide you through the movement, and your elbows should remain slightly bent at the top of the extension and your hips should remain in contact with the mat. Hold the up position for 15–30 seconds and then gently roll your upper body back to the floor.

Superman

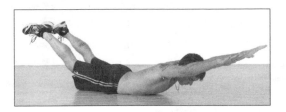

1 Lying face down on your stomach, extend your arms directly out in front of you and your legs behind you. Keep your knees straight as if you were flying.

2 In a slow and controlled manner, contract your erector spinae and raise your arms and legs about 6–8 inches off the floor. Hold for 5 seconds before lowering.

VARIATION: *This can also be done by holding a medicine ball between both hands. Use a very light medicine ball to start.*

In & Out

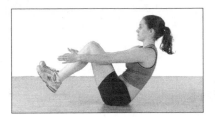

1 Lie flat on your back with your legs extended straight along the floor and your arms along your sides, palms down.

2 Lift your feet about 3 inches off the floor, bend your knees and bring your feet toward your butt while simultaneously lifting your arms off the floor and activating your abs to roll your upper body upward.

3 Continue raising your head and shoulders off the floor and bringing your hands past the outside of your knees while bringing your knees and chest together. At the top of the move, pause for 1–3 seconds.

Slowly return to start position. Be careful to "roll" your spine in a natural movement and let your shoulders and head lightly touch the floor.

Swoop & Touch

1 Lie flat on your back with your heels on the apex of a stability ball and knees bent 90 degrees. Completely extend both arms directly over your head and allow them to rest on the floor.

2 Swing your arms outward to each side as if you were making a snow angel on the floor and lift your shoulders and upper back off the floor as you reach your fingertips toward the ball. Keep your legs still and the ball in place as you complete the movement— you should be crunching your abs, not rolling the ball with your heels.

3 Touch the ball lightly and then reverse the movement, rolling your spine gently until your shoulders touch the floor. Lightly touch the back of your head to the floor.

That's 1 rep.

V-Sit

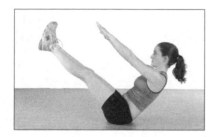

1 Lie flat on your back with your legs extended straight along the floor and your arms extended overhead on the floor with your biceps by your ears.

2 Contracting your abdominal muscles and keeping your legs straight, raise your legs and upper torso to form a "V." Your straight arms can be held parallel to your legs or alongside your ears. Hold the position for at least 3 seconds.

Slowly lower everything down without touching the ground with your heels or shoulders, then perform another rep.

Ab Crunch with Toe Touch

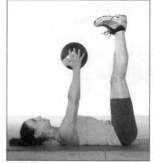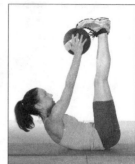

1 Lie face up on the floor with your legs straight and heels pointing at the ceiling so that your body is in an "L" position. Place the medicine ball on the center of your chest, with your hands on opposite sides of it to keep it in place. Press the ball straight up toward your toes.

2 Exhale and contract your abdominal muscles to slowly lift your head, arms and upper back off the floor in a controlled manner. Keep your upper back and neck straight and maintain your hand position on the ball through the movement. Push the medicine ball upward to touch the tips of your toes. Pause briefly.

Keeping your abs tight, inhale and return to the start position, lightly touching both shoulder blades to the floor. You may round your upper back slightly and roll your spine on the floor as you do so.

Mason Twist

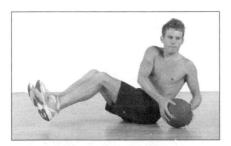

1 Sit on the floor with your knees comfortably bent, feet on the floor, arms bent 90 degrees, and hands holding a medicine ball or weight in front of your chest.

Lift your feet about 4–6 inches off the floor and balance your body weight on your posterior. Keep your core tight to protect your back.

2 While maintaining the same hip position, twist your entire torso at the waist and touch the ball to the floor on the left side of your body.

3 Rotate back to center, keeping your feet off the floor and maintaining your balance using the supporting core muscles. Then rotate to your right and touch the ball to the floor.

Return to center. This is 1 rep.

T-Twist

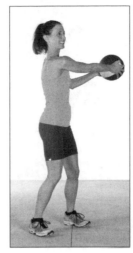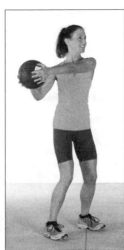

1 From an athletic position, hold a medicine ball at your waist with your arms extended.

2 Keeping your core tight and back straight, raise the medicine ball to shoulder height, directly in front of your torso with arms fully extended. Pause.

3 With your knees slightly bent, keep your hips facing forward while using your oblique muscles to rotate your upper body and the ball 90 degrees (or as far as you can go) to the right.

4 Slowly return to start position. Pause, then repeat to the other side. That's 1 rep.

Elephant Twist

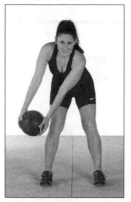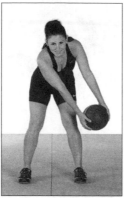

1 From an athletic position, hold a medicine ball in front of you with your arms extended. Bend forward at the waist 90 degrees so that the ball is hanging from your arms just above your feet.

2 Using your core, slowly twist your torso to the right 30 to 45 degrees (or as far as you can comfortably go) so that your arms and the ball form a straight line pointing at the ground outside of your right leg.

3 In a slow, controlled manner, straighten your torso and return the ball to the center position between your legs. Pause, then repeat to the left side.

Bring the ball back to center and lift the medicine ball back to start position by engaging your hamstrings and glutes to assist your lower back.

That's 1 rep.

Wood Chop

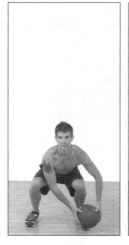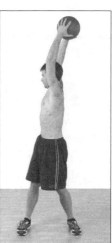

1 Stand tall with your feet shoulder-width apart, holding a medicine ball in front of you.

2 Lower your body into a squat until your knees are bent 90 degrees, and bring the ball down to touch your left foot.

3 Stand tall, twisting your torso to the right and lifting your arms straight up over your head. Your left shoulder should be in front and you should be looking to the right.

Repeat to the other side. That's 2 reps.

Flutter Kick

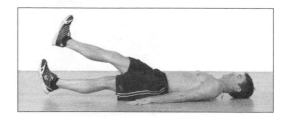

1 Lie flat on your back with your legs extended along the floor and your arms along your sides, palms down.

2 Contract your lower abdominal muscles and lift your feet 6 inches off the floor. Hold for 5 seconds. (You may flex or point your toes.)

3 While keeping your left foot in place, lift your right foot 6 inches higher (it should now be 12 inches off the floor). Hold for 5 seconds.

4 Simultaneously lower your right leg back to 6 inches off the floor while raising your left foot 6 inches higher. Hold for 5 seconds.

This counts as 2 reps.

Turkish Get-Up

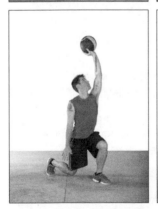 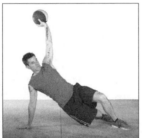

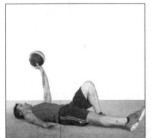 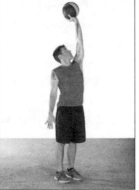

1 Lie face up on the floor and press a medicine ball to the ceiling with your left hand. Your right arm should be extended along the floor at about 45 degrees relative to your torso. Your right leg is extended straight out from your hip, toes pointing upward. Bend your left knee and bring your left heel as close to your butt as possible, with your toe rotated outward about 5–10 degrees.

2 Press your left hand higher while rolling your torso onto your right forearm, bending at the elbow and pressing your left heel into the floor to raise your left glute off the floor while rolling onto your right hip.

3 With your left hand still holding the medicine ball, press off the floor with your right forearm and hand to straighten your right arm and place your hand on the floor; press your hips upward to lift your butt off the floor. You're now supported by your left foot flat on the ground, the outside of your right foot and your right hand.

4 Bend your right knee and bring your right foot under your body, resting your weight on your right knee directly under your left hip. Push off with your right arm a little bit and rotate your torso back to square with your hips and align your knees under your hips, keeping your torso straight and perpendicular to the ground, left arm pressing the medicine ball directly overhead. Your body should look exactly like the lunge position with your left leg bent 90 degrees, foot flat on the floor, and your right leg 90 degrees with your toes and your right knee on the floor.

5 Pushing up through your left heel, straighten both knees and stand up, still keeping your left arm extended overhead with the medicine ball. Congratulations, that's exactly half of the exercise! Reverse the motion to return to start position.

Plank

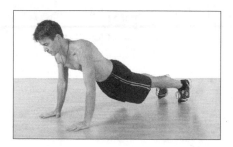

1 Place your hands on the ground approximately shoulder-width apart, making sure your fingers point straight ahead and your arms are straight but your elbows not locked. Step your feet back until your body forms a straight line from head to feet. Your feet should be about 6 inches apart with the weight in the balls of your feet. Engage your core to keep your spine from sagging; don't sink into your shoulders. Look at your watch and note the time—you're on the clock.

Lower to start position when time is reached.

VARIATION: *This can also be done with a medicine ball. Place both hands on top of the ball and roll it forward to position the ball directly under the center of your chest.*

Roll-Out

This is a subtle movement. The ball may move as little as an inch in either direction, though experienced athletes should shoot for more.

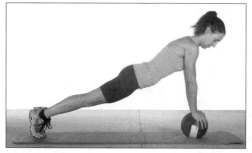

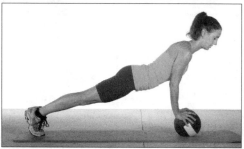

1 From your knees, place both hands on top of a medicine ball and roll it forward to position the ball directly under your sternum (the center of your chest). Straighten your legs, with the balls of your feet and toes in contact with the floor. Reposition your hands as needed to obtain a stable position. Engage your core and squeeze your glutes together to keep your spine erect and your body in a straight line from head to toe.

2 Using your forearms and hands, roll the ball forward (toward your head) as far as you can.

3 Bring it back to start position, then roll it backward (toward your feet) as far as you can before.

Return to start position.

Inchworm

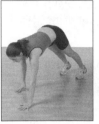 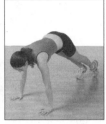 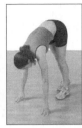

1 Stand with your feet about hip-width apart and fold over so that your hands touch the floor.

2 Keeping your hands firmly on the floor to balance your weight, walk your hands out in front of you one at a time until you're at the top of a push-up. Hold for 3 seconds.

3 Keeping your hands firmly on the floor to balance your weight, "walk" your feet toward your head by taking very small steps on your toes. Imagine that your lower legs are bound together and you can only bend your feet at each ankle. As you continue walking your feet toward your head, your butt will rise and your body will form an inverse "V." When you've stretched your hamstrings, glutes and calves as far as you can, hold that position for 3 seconds. That's 1 rep.

Bird Dog

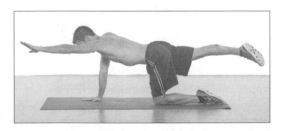

1 Get on your hands and knees with your legs bent 90 degrees, knees under your hips, toes on the floor and your hands on the floor directly below your shoulders. Keep your head and spine neutral; do not let your head lift or sag. Contract your abdominal muscles to prevent your back from sagging; keep your back flat from shoulders to butt for the entire exercise.

2 In one slow and controlled motion, simultaneously raise your right leg and left arm until they're on the same flat plane as your back. Your leg should be parallel to the ground, not raised above your hip; your arm should extend directly out from your shoulder and your biceps should be level with your ear. Hold this position for 3–5 seconds and then slowly lower your arm and leg back to start position.

That's 1 rep. Switch sides and repeat.

Side Plank

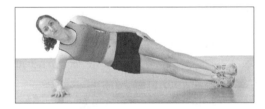

1 Lie on your side and stack your feet, hips and shoulders atop each other. Prop yourself up on your elbow, keeping it directly under your shoulder; your forearm should be completely on the ground, perpendicular to your body.

2 Engaging your core to keep your spine erect, lift your hips off the floor until you form a nice line from head to feet. Let your top arm rest along your side. Hold.

Slowly lower your hips to the floor. Repeat on the opposite side.

Sit-Up

If you have trouble keeping your feet on the ground, you can use a partner or a fixed object.

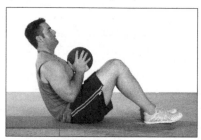

1 Lie face up on the floor with your knees bent about 90 degrees. Maintain proper curvature of your lower spine, not forcing it flat to touch the floor. Hold a medicine ball in the center of your chest, with your hands on opposite sides of the ball.

2 Exhale and contract your abdominal muscles to slowly lift your head, arms and upper back off the floor in a controlled manner. Keep your upper back and neck straight and maintain your hand position on the ball throughout the movement. Stop when your back is at about a 45-degree angle relative to the floor. Pause briefly.

Keeping your abs tight, inhale and return to the start position, lightly touching both shoulder blades to the floor. You may round your upper back slightly and roll your spine on the floor as you do so.

Crunch

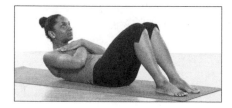

1 On a padded surface, lie face up with your knees bent to about 90 degrees your feet flat on the floor;

they should remain there during the entire movement. Rest your head, shoulders and back on the floor and maintain proper curvature of your lower spine, not allowing it to touch the floor. Cross your arms across your chest.

2 Exhale and contract your abdominal muscles to lift your head and shoulder blades off the floor in a controlled manner. Keep your upper back and neck straight and maintain the same position with your hands and arms throughout the movement. Pause briefly before slowly lowering your body to the floor.

Bicycle Crunch

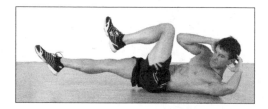

1 Lie flat on your back with your legs extended straight along the floor and your hands at both sides of your head, fingers touching your temples.

2 Raise your feet 6 inches off the floor while simultaneously contracting your rectus abdominis and lifting your upper back and shoulders off the floor. In one movement, bend your left knee and raise your left leg so that the thigh and shin are at 90 degrees; rotate your torso using your oblique muscles so that your right elbow touches the inside of your left knee.

3 Rotate your torso back to center and lower your upper body toward the floor, stopping before your shoulders touch.

4 Extend your left knee and return your foot to 6 inches off the floor and bend your right leg to 90 degrees. Contract your abs, rotate and touch your left elbow to the inside of your right knee. This is 2 reps.

Reverse Crunch

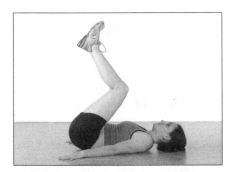

1 Lie flat on your back with your legs extended along the floor and your arms along your sides, palms down.

2 Contracting your lower abdominal muscles, lift your feet 4–6 inches off the floor, bend your knees and bring them in toward your chest. Be careful not to put excessive pressure on your lower back by bringing your hips off the floor. Pause when your glutes rise slightly off the mat.

3 Extend your legs and lower them until your feet are 4–6 inches off the floor.

Plank Row

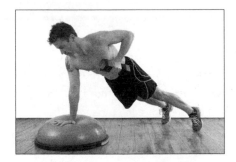

1 Get on your knees and place your right hand directly on the BOSU Balance Trainer's bull's-eye, right arm fully extended. Hold a dumbbell in your left hand. Lift your knees off the floor and extend your legs behind you with your feet wider than your shoulders. Keep your back flat and core engaged throughout the exercise.

2 Bend your left elbow and pull the dumbbell to your torso, pointing your elbow directly at the ceiling. Pause.

Return the dumbbell to start position. Complete half the required reps with your left hand rowing the weight, then switch hands.

Side Plank Fly

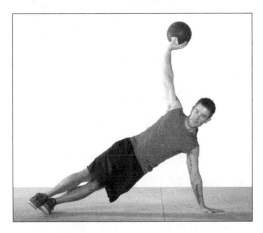

1 With your left arm supporting your upper body, rotate your entire body to the right, slowly raising your right hand and pressing the ball upward until your body forms a "T." Stack your feet on top of each other if you can (stop if you experience any knee instability), maintain a contracted core and keep your spine erect. Pause.

2 Slowly rotate your torso back to plank position, controlling the downward motion of the medicine ball by cradling it with your right hand, then placing it on the floor. Roll the ball to your left, switch hand positions and repeat. That's 1 rep.

T Push-Up

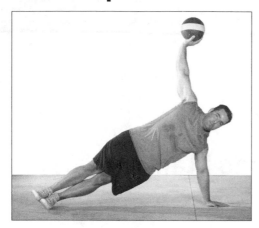

1 Assume a plank position (see page 136) with your right hand on the medicine ball and your left hand flat on the floor. Engage your core to keep your spine erect and keep your body in a straight line from head to toe.

2 Inhale as you lower your upper body toward the floor, stopping when your chest touches the back of your right hand.

3 Using your arms, chest, back and core, exhale and push off the floor to return to start position, gradually transitioning your weight to your left hand while sliding your right hand under the medicine ball (you'll be cupping it in order to lift it).

4 With your left arm supporting your upper body, rotate your entire body to the right, slowly raising your right hand and pressing the ball upward until your body forms a "T." Stack your feet on top of each other if you can (stop if you experience any knee instability), maintain a contracted core and keep your spine erect. Pause.

Slowly rotate your torso back to plank position, controlling the downward motion of the medicine ball by cradling it with your right hand, then placing it on the floor. Roll the ball to your left, switch hand positions and repeat. That's 1 rep.

Stability Ball Extension

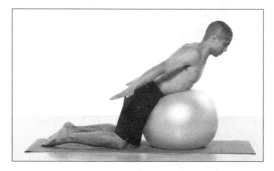

1 Kneeling on the floor, place a stability ball in front of you and lean your upper body forward so your torso rounds over the top of the ball. Roll forward about 2 inches while keeping the ball in contact with your thighs; your hips should now be at about a 100–110-degree angle.

2 Once you're positioned on the ball and stable, extend your arms back toward your hips with your palms facing downward. Contract the muscles of your lower back to raise your chest and sternum off the ball and straighten your back. Pause for 1–3 seconds and slowly return to the start position, trying not to bounce off the ball for each motion.

Hip Raise

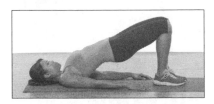

1 Lie on your back with your knees bent and feet flat on the floor, as close to your butt as possible. Extend your hands toward your hips and place your arms and palms flat on the floor at your sides.

2 Engage your abdominal muscles to keep your core tight, and exhale while you press your feet into the floor and raise your hips and lower back up, forming a straight line from your sternum to your knees. Do not push your hips too high or arch your back. Hold this position for 3–5 seconds, and then inhale and slowly return to the start position.

Weighted Hip Thrust

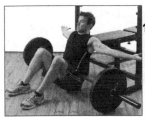 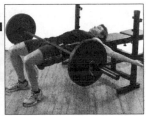

Sit on the floor and position a bench behind your upper back so that your shoulder blades make contact with the edge of the bench. Place your feet flat on the floor and lay a weighted bar, medicine ball or weight plate across your hips or at the very top of your pelvis (make sure the weight doesn't roll or shift to hit you in the genitals). Extend your arms out to your sides, parallel to the floor, or rest them on your chest.

2 Driving through your heels, use your hamstrings, hips and glutes to raise your pelvis toward the ceiling and slide your upper back onto the bench. Your body should form a straight line from head to knees. Squeeze your abs and glutes, and brace your lower back to hold the flat position for 3–5 seconds. In a slow and controlled manner, lower your butt back to the ground, carefully sliding your upper back off the bench.

Hanging Leg Raise

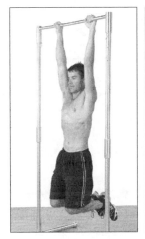 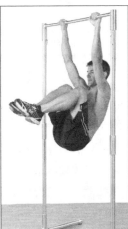

1 Grab an overhead bar with your preferred grip and hang from the bar with your arms fully extended but elbows not locked. For this exercise, count 3 seconds up, hold 1–3 seconds, and then 3 seconds down.

2 Contracting your abdominal muscles, slowly bring your knees up toward your chest while keeping your torso as close to vertical as possible. Don't lean back during the movement or swing between reps.

Lower your legs in the same slow manner.

Marching Twist

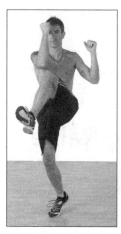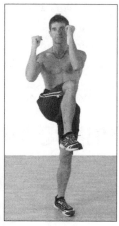

1 Stand tall with your feet shoulder-width apart. Bring your arms in front of you and bend your elbows 90 degrees.

2 Twist your torso to the left and raise your left knee to your right elbow.

3 Repeat with your right knee and left elbow. A little hop with the bottom foot helps you keep your momentum going from leg to leg.

That's 2 reps.

Jumping Jacks

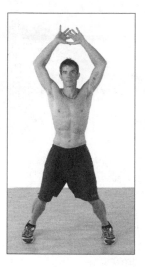

1 Stand tall with your feet together and arms extended along your sides, palms facing forward.

2 Jump 6–12 inches off the ground and simultaneously spread your feet apart an additional 20–30 inches while extending your hands directly overhead.

Jump 6–12 inches off the ground and return your hands and feet to the start position.

Skater Hop

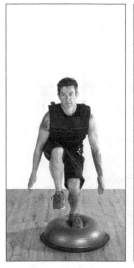 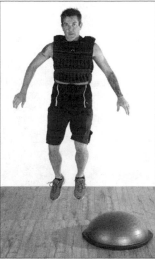

1 Stand with your left foot directly on the bull's-eye and your right foot on the floor beside the BOSU Balance Trainer. Find a stable position and engage your core. Your arms should hang along your sides. Wearing a weighted vest intensifies the work.

2 Shifting your weight onto your left foot and balancing on the apex of the dome, lift your right foot off the floor and bend your knee 90 degrees (about hip level). You may tap the toes of your elevated leg to the ground for balance. As your balance and stability improve, work toward raising the knee of your "up" leg toward your chest.

3 Bend your left knee, rotate your hips back slightly and sink straight down into a squat position (page 148). Keep your left shin vertical and don't let your knee buckle to the right or left; place your right foot down and re-start if you lose your balance. *Note:* You'll most likely not be able to perform a full squat at first; descend as far as you can while maintaining good form. You should be able to go deeper as you progress in your training.

4 Swing both arms forward and in one explosive move straighten your left leg and hop directly to your right, landing with your right foot first and then your left. Align both feet parallel to each other, with knees slightly bent to absorb the impact of landing.

Stand up and return to start position. That's 1 rep. Repeat with your right foot on the bull's-eye.

Side Hop

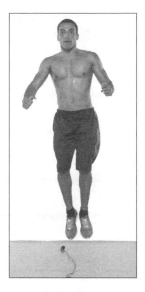

1 Stand parallel to some kind of flat marker so that it's about 10 inches away from your right foot. Bend your knees, crouch at your waist and swing your arms down by your sides and prepare to jump over the marker.

2 Leaning slightly to the right, extend your legs forcefully and jump to your right as high as you can and land with your left foot approximately 10 inches to the right of the marker. Bend your knees and land softy on the balls of your feet in a controlled manner.

Immediately after landing, jump over the marker to your left, landing with your right foot approximately 10 inches to the left of the marker. That's 1 rep.

Mountain Climbers

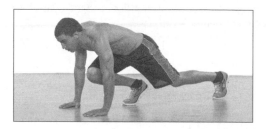

1 Assume the top position of a push-up with your hands directly under your shoulders and toes on the ground. Keep your core engaged and your body in a straight line from head to feet.

2 Lift your right toe slightly off the ground, bring your right knee to your chest and place your right foot on the ground under your body.

3 With a very small hop from both toes, extend your right foot back to start position and at the same time bring your left knee to your chest and place your left foot on the ground under your body.

That's 2 reps. Continue switching, making sure to keep your hips low.

Burpee

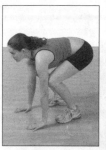 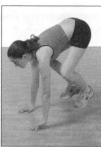 

1 Stand tall with your back erect, feet shoulder-width apart and toes rotated slightly outward. Shift your hips backward and "sit back" for the squat, keeping your head up and bending your knees. Lean your weight forward and place your hands on the floor, inside, outside or in front of your feet—whichever is more comfortable and gives you a nice, stable base.

2 Kick your feet straight back so that you're now in a push-up start position, forming a nice line from your head to your feet. Keep your core tight to maintain an erect spine.

3 Now simultaneously bend your knees and bring them toward your chest in order to plant your feet underneath you. You should end up back in the bottom position of a squat. Take a quick breath.

4 Swing your arms straight overhead, exhale and push off from your feet to jump straight up in the air as high as possible. Land with your knees slightly bent to absorb the impact. That's 1 rep.

VARIATION: *Rather than jump your feet forward/ backward, walk them in and out (see Inchworm on page 137).*

Bizarro Burpee

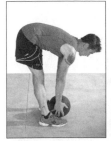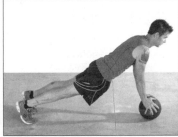

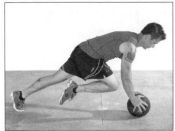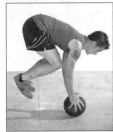

1 From an athletic position, hold a medicine ball at your waist with your arms extended. Keeping your lower back straight and knees slightly bent, bend at the waist and lower the medicine ball to the ground between your feet, tracking close to your legs the entire way down.

2 Place both hands securely on the top of the medicine ball, squat down and kick your feet out behind you, extending your legs and placing the balls of your feet and toes on the floor for balance. A snapshot of this position should look exactly like a medicine ball plank.

3 With your upper body balanced on the medicine ball, lift your right foot, bend your right knee and pull it up toward your right elbow, stopping before you make contact.

4 Extend your right knee and place your foot back on the floor. Now bring your left knee to your left elbow.

5 Extend your left leg back into the plank position.

6 Bending at the waist, hop both feet back on each side of the medicine ball, straighten your legs and lift the medicine ball back to the start position, engaging your hamstrings and glutes to assist your lower back to extend your waist.

Burpee with Overhead Press & Lunge

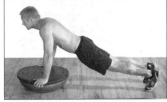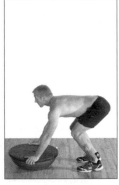

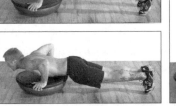

1 Stand approximately half a body's length behind the BOSU Balance Trainer, dome-side down. Smoothly jump your feet backward, landing softly on your toes. Simultaneously drop your upper body toward the BOSU Balance Trainer, softly landing your hands on the outside rim of the flat base, and grab the handles.

2 Keeping your core tight and back flat, perform a push-up by slowly lowering your chest to touch the flat side.

3 Still gripping the handles, use your arms and chest to explosively push your upper body away from the BOSU Balance Trainer while bending at the waist and jumping your feet forward, back under your body. Land with your knees bent in a semi-squatting position (approximately 45 degrees).

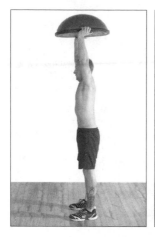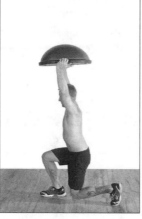

4 Stand up straight, lifting the BOSU Balance Trainer and pressing it directly above your head.

5 Step forward with your right foot and lower your left knee straight down in a lunge; stop when both knees are bent 90 degrees. Keep your back straight and arms fully extended.

6 Press off your right foot and left toes to return to standing, squat and lower the BOSU Balance Trainer back to the floor. That's 1 rep. Repeat with other leg.

Thruster

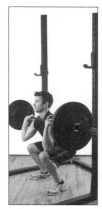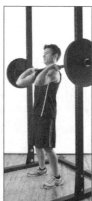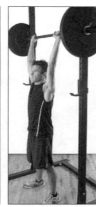

1 In a squat rack or cage, position an Olympic bar just below shoulder height. Step into the bar, positioning

it on the natural shelf just above your chest and below your collarbone. Using your fingers (not your palms), hold the bar in position above your chest. Your elbows should be pointing straight forward or slightly up, if possible. The bigger your biceps, the harder the positioning is. The higher you can get your elbows, the more stable you will be.

2 Lift the bar out of the rack and step back or forward one step. Engage your core. Sit back slightly and lower your body in a typical squat. Your torso should be completely upright to support the bar on the front of your body rather than the back of your body. Core engagement is key.

3 Pause at the bottom, then push through your glutes and return to start position.

4 Take a deep breath, squeeze your glutes and core, and tuck your tailbone to provide a strong, stable base. Press the bar in a straight line directly overhead. Once the bar has passed the top of your head, press your upper body and head forward so the bar is directly overhead and the insides of your elbows are about laterally even with your ears. When the bar reaches its apex, your entire body should be in a strong, stable position; your legs, glutes, core, shoulders, upper back and arms should all be activated to keep the weight in place.

5 Slowly lower the bar, tilting your head back and controlling the bar's decent until it softly touches your collarbone. (Softly! Your collarbone, or clavicle, can be broken by less than 10 pounds of force!) Exhale.

Ball Thruster

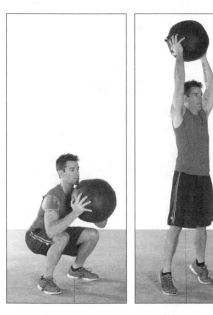

1 From an athletic position, hold a medicine ball to your chest with your arms bent.

2 Bend at the hips and lower your body into a goblet squat (page 148) until your knees are bent at least 90 degrees. Pause.

3 While pushing straight up from your heels back to standing, press the medicine ball directly overhead by rotating your shoulders forward and extending your arms; your biceps should finish in line with your ears. Don't lock your knees at the top of the exercise. Keep your core flexed throughout the movement and don't arch your back when you lift the ball overhead. Pause.

Carefully reverse the motion and return the ball back to your chest.

Wall Ball

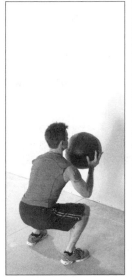
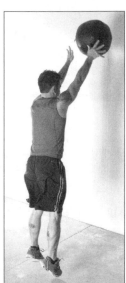

1 From an athletic position facing a wall about 2 feet away, hold a medicine ball to your chest with your arms bent. Look up and pick a spot on the wall that's at least 8 feet above the floor—that'll be your target to hit with the ball.

2 Bend at the hips and lower your body into a goblet squat (page 148) until your knees are bent at least 90 degrees. Pause.

3 Push straight up from your heels back to standing while explosively pressing and tossing the medicine ball upward and slightly forward to the target on the wall; your biceps should finish in line with your ears. Your weight should transfer to your forefeet as you explode upward, and your feet should leave the ground.

Land with your knees bent, keeping an eye on the ball the entire time. Catch the ball with your elbows bent then carefully return the ball back to your chest, making sure not to bonk yourself in the head, nose or chin.

Squat

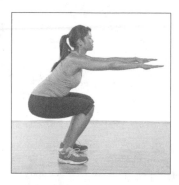

1 Stand tall with your feet shoulder-width apart and toes pointed slightly outward, about 11 and 1 o'clock. Raise your arms until they're parallel to the floor.

2 Bend at the hips and knees and "sit back" just a little bit as if you were about to sit directly down into a chair. Keep your head up, eyes forward and arms out in front of you for balance. As you descend, contract your glutes while your body leans forward slightly so that your shoulders are almost in line with your knees. Your knees should not extend past your toes and your weight should remain between the heel and the middle of your feet—do not roll up on the balls of your feet. Stop when your knees are at 90 degrees and your thighs are parallel to the floor. If you feel your weight is on your toes or heels, adjust your posture and balance until your weight is in the middle of your feet.

Push straight up from your heels back to the start position. Don't lock your knees at the top of the exercise.

Goblet Squat

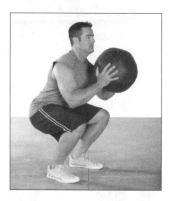

1 From an athletic position, hold a medicine ball to your chest with your arms bent.

2 Keeping your head up, eyes forward and core tight, bend at the hips and knees and "sit back" to perform the squat.

Keeping the medicine ball at chest height, push straight up from your heels back to the start position. Don't lock your knees at the top of the exercise.

Back Squat

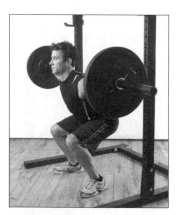

1 Place the bar in a stable, somewhat comfortable position across your upper back at shoulder height. Stand centered under the bar and place your hands 6–8 inches wider than your shoulders on the bar in an overhand grip. Your knees should be slightly bent to allow you to get under the bar. Place your feet approximately shoulder-width apart and straighten your legs to lift the weight off the rack. Carefully step forward just enough to clear the bar of the J-cups. Stand up straight with your shoulders back (your chest should be as wide as possible) and keep your chin up, head looking straight ahead. Take a deep breath and tighten your abdominal muscles to stabilize your core and protect your back during the descent.

2 Rotate your hips backward and slowly perform a squat, keeping your head and chest up. Do not let your knees bow in or you can cause some serious damage. If you cannot keep your knees in the proper line, you are trying to squat too much weight and are in danger of spraining or tearing your medial collateral ligament (MCL).

Breathe out and drive your upper body straight up through your heels back to start position. Do not bounce at the bottom or the top, and be extremely careful not to snap-lock and potentially hyperextend your knees at the top.

Front Squat

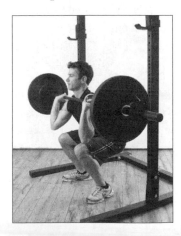

1 In a squat rack or cage, position an Olympic bar just below shoulder height. Step into the bar, positioning it on the natural shelf just above your chest and below your collarbone. Using your fingers (not your palms), hold the bar in position above your chest. Your elbows should be pointing straight forward or slightly up, if possible. The bigger your biceps, the harder the positioning is. The higher you can get your elbows, the more stable you will be.

2 Lift the bar out of the rack and take one step back. Engage your core. Sit back slightly and lower your body in a typical squat. Your torso should be completely upright to support the bar on the front of your body rather than the back of your body. Core engagement is key.

Pause at the bottom, then push through your glutes and return to start position.

Single-Leg Squat

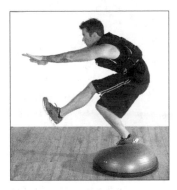

1 Stand with both feet directly on either side of the bull's-eye of a BOSU Balance Trainer. Find a stable position and engage your core.

2 Keeping your knee over your toe, bend your right knee and lower your body until your glutes drop as close as possible to parallel. Do not lean forward. Pause.

Push up with your right leg, returning to start position.

Lunge

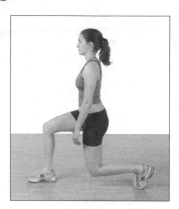

1 Stand tall with your feet shoulder-width apart and your arms hanging at your sides.

2 Take a large step forward with your right foot, bend both knees and drop your hips straight down until both knees are bent 90 degrees. Your left knee should almost be touching the ground and your left toes are on the ground behind you. Keep your core engaged and your back, neck and hips straight at all times during this movement.

Pushing up with your right leg, straighten both knees and return to starting position. Repeat with the other leg.

Jump Lunge

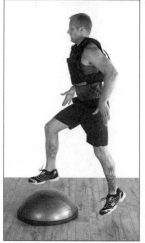 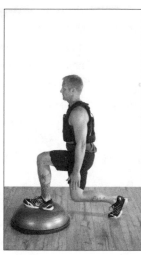

1 Stand with a BOSU Balance Trainer approximately a stride's length in front of you. Stand upright with your hands along your sides.

2 Keeping your left leg in place, stride forward with your right leg, bending your right knee slightly. Land your right mid-foot directly on the bull's-eye, keeping your right knee behind your toes.

3 Continue the stride's natural descent until your left knee almost touches the ground.

4 Explode up through your right heel and mid-foot and switch leg positions at the peak of your jump. You should use enough force to leave the ground with both feet.

5 Land your left mid-foot directly on the bull's-eye, aiming to keep your left knee behind your toes.

Continue the stride's natural descent until your right knee almost touches the ground. That's 1 rep.

Lunge with Twist

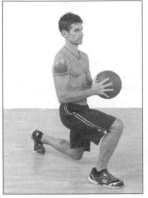 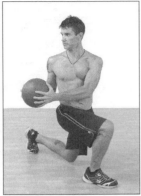

1 Stand tall with your feet shoulder-width apart and both hands on opposite sides of a medicine ball, elbows slightly bent.

2 Keeping the ball directly in front of you, step forward (or backward) with your right foot to start the lunge motion. As you lower your hips, twist your core and swing the ball laterally to your right until both knees are bent 90 degrees and your arms are extended and holding the medicine ball to the right, 90 degrees from where you started.

Return to start position. That's 1 rep. Repeat to the other side.

Lunge with Biceps Curl

1 Stand tall with your hands at your sides holding dumbbells. Keep your core tight.

2 Step forward with your right leg into a lunge (your knee shouldn't extend past your toes), slowly lowering your left knee toward the floor.

3 As you lower, curl the dumbbells. You should finish the curl at about the same time as you finish the lunge.

4 Push up through your right heel and return to the starting position with your arms by your sides. Alternate legs.

Bulgarian Split Squat

1 Holding a dumbbell in each hand, stand with your right foot approximately 12 inches in front of you and your left foot balanced on a bench behind you. Balance on both feet equally.

2 With your weight on your right heel, descend until your left knee touches the floor.

3 Push through your right heel and return to start position.

Repeat, then switch legs.

Toe Touch

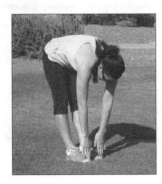

1 Stand with your feet approximately shoulder-width apart and back straight. Lift your arms directly above your head with your palms facing forward. Reach up as high as you can.

2 Hinge at your waist and, keeping your arms overhead and back as straight as possible, lower your upper torso as one unit to bring your head toward your knees. Try to touch your toes with your fingertips. Do not bounce or grab your ankles in an attempt to pull your upper body farther down. Hold in the down position for 5 seconds.

Slowly return to the start position with your arms extended over your head. Repeat, each time trying to stretch a little farther than the previous repetition.

Good Morning

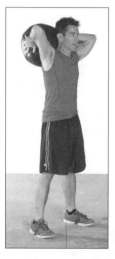
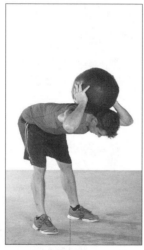

1 From an athletic position, lift the medicine ball over your head and rest it carefully on the top of your back, on your spine just below your neck. Do not place the ball on your neck—the added weight on your cervical vertebrae can cause you to arch your neck, causing pain and discomfort. Steady the ball in position with your hands and bring your elbows in toward your head.

2 Keeping your core tight and back flat, bend forward at the waist until your torso is parallel to the floor. Pause.

Slowly return to the start position.

Deadlift

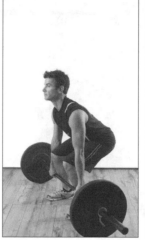
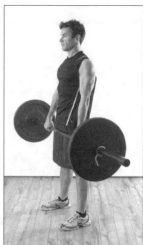

1 Starting with an Olympic bar on the floor, choose a light weight and place an equal number and weight of plates on either end. Position your feet shoulder-width apart with your toes under the bar and your shins very close to the bar. Grasp the bar with either an overhand or mixed grip (one underhand, one overhand) a few inches outside of your legs in relation to the bar. Push your hips directly back slightly, lift your chest and keep your chin up with your head looking directly in front of you. Do not hunch your shoulders or lean forward; your back should be primarily straight with a natural curve.

2 Take a deep breath, and then drive through your heels and extend your legs to lift the bar straight up toward the top of your thighs while rising to a standing position. Finish the move by pressing your hips forward, aligning your shoulders, hips, knees and ankles in a straight line. Do not lean back at the top of the movement, this will put undue stress on your lower back.

Slowly and carefully reverse the move to lower the bar to the floor. Do not bend over and place the bar on the ground—the bar should follow the exact same path as it did while you were raising it. Do not drop the bar from the top or you'll be missing out on half of the exercise!

Romanian Deadlift

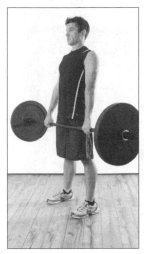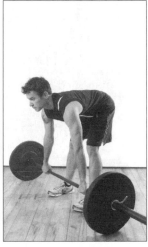

1 Grasping a barbell with an overhand grip, stand upright with the barbell at leg level, arms fully extended. Keep the core, lower back, glutes and hips tight and focused.

2 Never relaxing the core, lower back, glutes or hips, slowly lower the bar toward the ground, not quite touching the ground

Pause, then return to start position.

VARIATION: *This can also be done with a medicine ball. From an athletic position, hold a medicine ball at your waist with your arms fully extended. Bend at the waist to lower the ball as close as you can to your legs as you descend.*

Single-Leg Deadlift

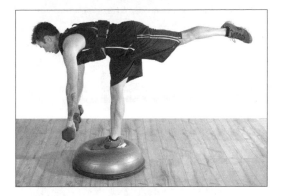

1 Holding a dumbbell in each hand at your sides, stand with both feet on either side of the bull's-eye of a BOSU Balance Trainer. Find a stable position. Engage your core.

2 Lift your left foot, fully extend your right leg and bend at the waist. Simultaneously lower your upper body and raise your left leg behind you until your entire backside, all the way from your left heel to your head, forms one straight line. Pause.

Pull through your right hamstring and glutes to return to start position.

Repeat, then switch sides.

Clean

1 Just like the deadlift, start with a barbell on the floor touching your shins, feet parallel and hip-width apart. Hands should grasp the barbell just outside your legs. Keep your head up, core tight and shoulders back. These cues should give you a straight back from head to tail.

2 Pull the bar up and off the floor by extending your hips and knees. As the bar reaches your knees, pull through your shoulders while keeping the barbell close to your thighs.

3 When the barbell passes mid-thigh, jump upward, extending your body. Shrug your shoulders and pull the barbell upward, allowing your elbows to flex out to the sides but keeping the bar close to your body.

4 Now actively pull your body under the bar, rotating your elbows around the bar. Catch the bar on your shoulders just as you would position for a front squat (page 149).

Calf Raise

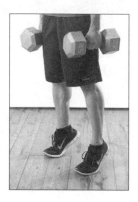

1 Holding a barbell or two dumbbells, lift the weight toward your waist and hold with your arms fully extended.

2 With your legs approximately shoulder-width apart and your toes pointed forward, press through the balls of your feet and raise your entire body and weight straight up. Maintain your balance on the balls of your feet and squeeze your calves to hold the "up" position for 1–3 seconds.

Slowly lower your heels back down to the floor.

Linear Reactive Step-Up

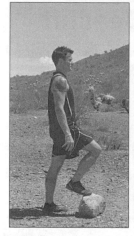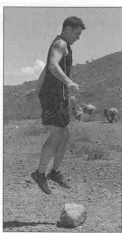

1 Stand 12–18 inches in front of a bench or object 18–24 inches tall that can hold your weight; have your hands at your sides and feet shoulder-width apart.

2 Step up with your right foot as if you were climbing a step and place it flat on top of the bench, leaving your left foot on the ground.

3 Push down with your right foot on top of the bench and jump up as high as you can using only the strength of your right leg. Your left leg should not be pushing off at all; this exercise works one leg at a time to develop explosive jumping power. Let your arms swing naturally at your sides as you jump.

4 Switch legs in mid-air by bringing your right foot backward and left foot forward at the apex of your jump. Your left foot will land on top of the bench and your right foot on the ground.

As soon as your left foot lands on the bench, immediately jump again using only the strength of your left leg.

That's 2 reps.

Step-Up with Dumbbell Curl

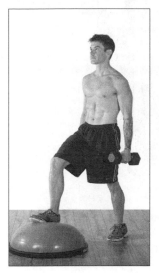 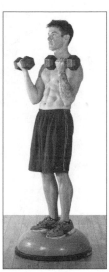

1 With the BOSU Balance Trainer approximately half a stride's length in front of you, stand upright with a dumbbell in each hand, arms fully extended at your sides. Step on the bull's-eye one foot at a time.

2 Bring your elbows in toward your sides and rotate your hands so that your palms face upward. Contracting your abs to keep your spine straight and keeping your upper arms next to your torso, slowly raise the weights toward your shoulders.

Box Jump

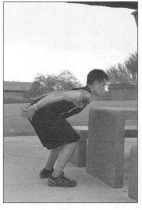 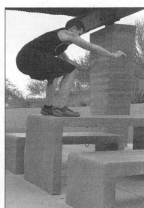

1 Start by standing 12–18 inches in front of a box or bench that's 24–36 inches tall and can hold your weight. Keep your hands at your sides and feet shoulder-width apart.

2 Initiate the jump by dropping your hips and bending at the waist in a squat movement, but only about half as deep. Swing your arms back and shift your weight toward the front of your feet.

3 Extend your hips, swing your arms forward, and push off from your feet to jump as high as you can toward the center top of the box. Land softly on the box with your knees bent to absorb the shock.

Step off to either side of the box, placing a hand on the edge of the box if necessary to keep your balance. Don't jump backward off the box.

Push-Up

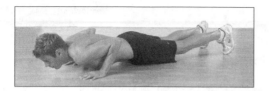

1 Place your hands on the ground approximately shoulder-width apart, making sure your fingers point straight ahead and your arms are straight but your elbows not locked. Step your feet back until your body forms a straight line from head to feet. Your feet should be about 6 inches apart with the weight in the balls of your feet. Engage your core to keep your spine from sagging; don't sink into your shoulders.

2 Inhale as you lower your torso to the ground and focus on keeping your elbows as close to your sides as possible, stopping when your elbows are at a 90 degree angle or your chest is 1–2 inches from the floor.

Exhale and return to start position.

VARIATION: *This can also be done by placing both hands on either side of a medicine ball. Lower your upper body to the ball before pushing back up.*

Pull-Up

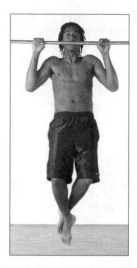

1 Grip the horizontal bar with your palms facing away from you and your arms fully extended. Your hands should be slightly wider than your shoulders. Your feet should not touch the floor during this exercise. Let all of your weight settle in position but do not relax your shoulders—this may cause them to overstretch.

2 Squeeze your shoulder blades together, look up at the bar, exhale and pull your chin up toward the bar by driving your elbows toward the floor. It's very important to keep your shoulders back and chest up during the entire movement. Pull yourself up in a controlled manner until the bar is just above the top of your chest.

3 Inhale and slowly lower yourself back down. Don't lock your elbows, swing your feet or "bounce" at the bottom of the movement before starting the upward movement.

Chin-Up

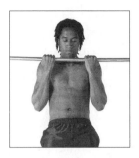

1 Perform the pull-up with your palms facing you.

Single-Arm Curl & Overhead Press

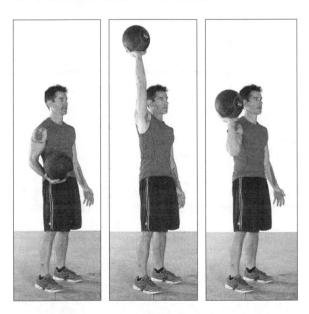

1 From an athletic position, hold a medicine ball in your right hand, with your arm bent 90 degrees and your elbow and upper arm against your side, as if you were a waiter holding a plate of food in front of you.

2 Flex your biceps and raise the ball to your shoulder so your fingers are nearly touching your shoulder.

3 Press the ball directly overhead in a slow and controlled manner. Pause.

Return the ball to your side. Flip the medicine ball to your left hand and repeat with your left hand. That's 1 rep.

Overhead Press

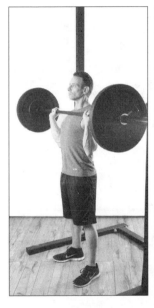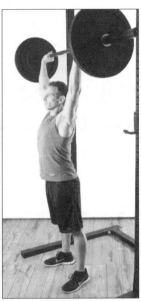

1 The bar should be positioned on a squat rack at shoulder height. It's recommended that you practice this exercise with no weight until you're familiar with the proper form. Grip the bar with an overhand grip just outside your shoulders. Rotate your elbows so they're under the bar, pointing directly away from your torso. Raise your chest and keep your head looking straight forward. You'll need to tilt your head back a little bit so the bar can clear your chin when you press the bar up. Unrack the bar and take a small step backward or forward (depending on your rack setup or preference) so the bar can clear the rack when you press it. Your feet should be even with each other and shoulder-width apart.

2 Take a deep breath, squeeze your glutes and core, and tuck your tailbone to provide a strong, stable base. Press the bar in a straight line directly overhead. Once the bar has passed the top of your head, press your upper body and head forward so the bar is directly overhead and the inside of your elbows are about laterally even with your ears. When the bar reaches its apex, your entire body should be in a strong, stable position; your legs, glutes, core, shoulders, upper back and arms should all be activated to keep the weight in place.

Overhead Press & Triceps Extension

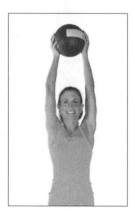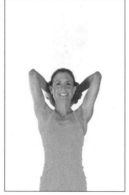

1 From an athletic position, hold a medicine ball to your chest with your arms bent.

2 Press the medicine ball directly overhead until your biceps are in line with your ears. Pause.

3 Slowly lower the ball behind your head while keeping your upper arms in line with your ears. Stop before the ball touches your upper back. Pause.

Raise the ball back overhead and carefully return to the start position.

Barbell Curl

This can be done with either a straight bar or an EZ curl bar. If you vary your hand position on the EZ bar, you can target different areas of the biceps and work the entire muscle.

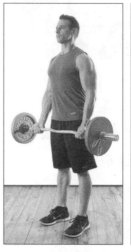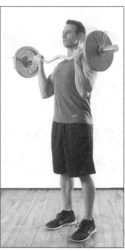

1 Grasp a barbell with an underhand grip. Lock your elbows either in place or to your hips/sides.

2 Raise the bar in an arc toward your shoulders, never fully reaching your shoulders. Stop when the biceps aren't doing the work anymore.

Pause, then slowly lower the bar to the start position.

Barbell Row

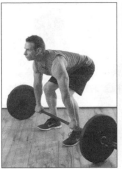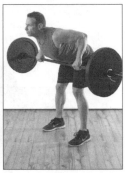

1 Place a barbell on the floor and position yourself over it. With your knees slightly bent and your back straight, bend forward at the waist until your back is approximately parallel with the ground. Reach down and grasp the barbell with an overhand grip and arms fully extended.

2 Using primarily your upper back, not your arms, pull the bar to your waist or lower torso. To activate your back more than your arms, mentally focus on squeezing your back and shoulder blades together as tightly as possible. You'll naturally use some arms, but the key is to minimize their involvement!

Pause, then return to the start position with your arms fully extended.

1-Arm Dumbbell Row

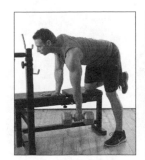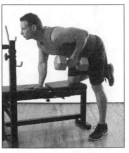

1 Position yourself on a flat bench with your left knee and left hand on the bench for support. Place your

right leg slightly back on the ground for support. Grasp a dumbbell with your right hand directly beneath your right shoulder.

2 Pull the dumbbell to your side until it makes contact with your waist. Pause, then return to start position. Don't put the dumbbell back on the ground.

Continue until all reps are complete, then repeat on your left side.

Dumbbell Shrug

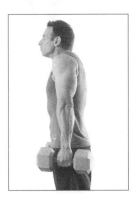

1 Grasp two dumbbells of the same weight. Hold them by your sides with your shoulders relaxed. Lean forward at the hips a bit, letting the weights hang just in front of you.

2 Flex your traps and pull your shoulders through your back. In other words, shrug. Pause at the top, then slowly lower to the start position, but never fully relax your shoulders.

Dip

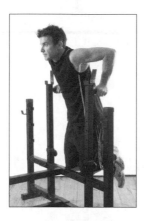

1 Step between two dip bars that are about shoulder-width apart. Non-parallel bars allow you to find a hand position (rotated in or out) and a width that's more comfortable. Grip the top of the bars securely and extend your arms completely with your body leaning about 5 degrees forward.

2 Lower your body in a controlled manner by bending your arms at the elbows. Be cautious of elbow or shoulder pain and adjust your positioning to lessen any strain. When your upper arms and forearms are roughly 90 degrees in relation to each other, your upper arms are parallel to the dip bar or your feel a deep stretch in your chest or shoulders, pause your descent.

Drive your hands back down toward your knees by using your triceps to return your arms to a fully extended position.

Triceps Kickback

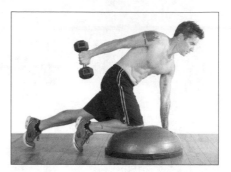

1 Start with your right knee on the dome of a BOSU Balance Trainer and your left hand supporting your weight either on the ground or the edge of the BOSU. Extend your left leg behind you with both toes on the ground for balance. Grasp the dumbbell with your right hand and raise it to your right hip.

2 Extend your elbow and press the dumbbell directly behind you by engaging your triceps. Don't rotate your shoulder; try to limit rotation of your torso. Pause.

3 Return to the start position.

Finish the desired reps and repeat on the opposite side.

Shoulder Raise

Shoulder raises should be done both to the sides and to the front. We recommend one full set to the sides followed by one full set to the front. Do not go heavy, but instead use lighter weights and slow, controlled motions.

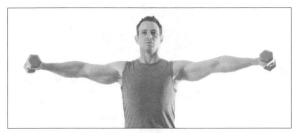

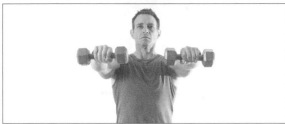

1 Grasp two dumbbells at your sides using an overhand grip, with the insides of your fists facing your body and thumbs roughly adjacent to your upper thighs.

2 Raise them away from your body to the sides and pause for 1–3 seconds when the weights are level with your shoulders. Then lower slowly to your sides. Repeat until you've completed half of the given reps for a workout before moving on to step 3.

3 Bring the dumbbells around toward the front of your body, with your palms facing the fronts of your hips. Your elbows should be slightly bent, core engaged to keep your back straight, knees slightly bent in an athletic posture.

4 Raise your arms directly in front of your body until the weights are at shoulder level. Your arms should be straight but your elbows not in a fully locked-out position. Pause for 1–3 seconds, then lower slowly back to start position.

Repeat steps 3–4 for the remainder of the required reps for a workout.

Chest Fly

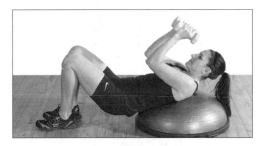

1 Lying on the dome of a BOSU Balance Trainer, position your shoulder blades so they're approximately on either side of the bull's-eye of the BOSU. Grasp a dumbbell in each hand with an overhand grip, bend both elbows approximately 90 degrees, and position your arms in line with your torso. The weights should be slightly above shoulder height with your inner arms and palms facing the ceiling. Raise your buttocks off the ground for the entire movement; keep your core tight in order to stabilize your back.

2 Keeping your elbows bent and your wrists in a locked position, engage your pectoral muscles to lift the weights—slowly swing them in an arc together directly over your sternum. Pause when your palms are facing each other and the weights are gently touching. Squeeze your chest together during the movement and especially when the weights are above your torso. Pause.

Slowly return to the start position.

Reverse Fly

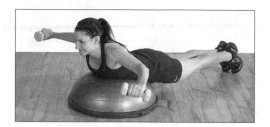

1 Lie face-down on top of a BOSU Balance Trainer dome with the bull's-eye centered on your torso slightly below your chest. Extend your legs and place your toes on the floor for balance. Grasp dumbbells in each hand with an overhand grip and place them on the floor, your arms nearly extended out on both sides of your shoulders. Squeeze your glutes to help brace your core. *Note:* Your elbows should be bent slightly, about 140–160 degrees relative to your upper arm.

2 Keeping your back straight and arms flat (don't rotate your forearms relative to your upper arms), lift the weights straight up off the floor using the large muscles of your upper back by squeezing your shoulder blades together. Pause at the top.

Lower slowly back to the start position.

Bench Press

Start with a broomstick or unweighted Olympic bar and practice proper technique throughout the entire movement before you add any weight at all. Oh, and find a spotter.

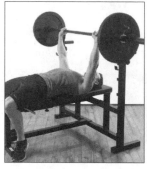 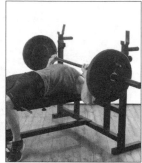

1 Check the bar position on the rack. When you lie under the bar you should be able to extend your elbows completely when you lift the bar off the safety pegs. You should never be raising the bar and moving it forward away from the safety supports with bent elbows. Lie back on the bench with your feet flat on the floor as wide as you comfortably can. Your heels should be solidly planted and very stable. If your legs are too short to be securely flat on the floor, slide a couple of 45-pound plates under your feet. Squeeze your shoulder blades together and broaden your chest.

Grip the bar and tightly tuck your elbows toward your sides and keep them as close to your body as you can during the entire movement.

2 Press the bar straight up off the safety pegs and extend your elbows into a locked position before moving the weight directly over your sternum. Do not unrack and descend the bar in one movement; the lateral momentum and possible overcompensation can cause the bar to fall on your ribcage or toward your neck or head. Be extremely careful and deliberate when you unrack the weight; extend your arms and get the bar on the right plane straight up, about 1–2 inches below your nipples or even with the bottom of your sternum.

3 Inhale, and in a controlled manner, lower the bar until it touches your chest.

4 Press the bar directly up in a straight line back to start position using your chest, arms and even the heels of your feet. Keep your glutes on the bench, shoulder blades retracted and chest up throughout the entire fluid movement as you breathe out. Extend your arms fully such that your elbows are straight and the weight is stable above you.

5 Carefully re-rack the bar when all the reps are complete.

Incline Bench Press

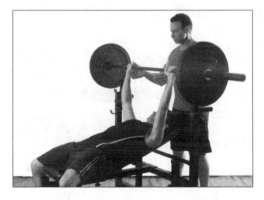

1 Set the bench angle between 20 and 40 degrees. The steeper the angle (or the higher the head portion of the bench), the more you'll be activating your shoulder muscles while using less of your chest.

Sit on the seat area of the bench and place both feet firmly on the ground on either side of the bench to form a stable, wide stance. Lie back on the bench and squeeze your shoulder blades together. Grip the bar and tuck your elbows in. Keep them as close to your sides as possible throughout the movement. Breathe in, extend your elbows and press the bar

straight up from the safety pegs. Carefully bring the bar directly over your upper chest and pause.

2 In a controlled manner, lower the bar to your chest and then drive it straight up.

3 Carefully re-rack the bar when all reps are complete.

VARIATION: *This can also be done by holding two dumbbells.*

Landmine

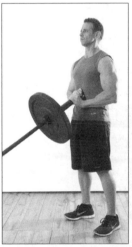 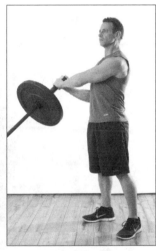

1 Place a 45-pound plate flat on the floor and position one end of a full-size Olympic bar in the plate's center hole on a 45-degree angle so that the tip of the bar is held in place, or in the corner of a room so the bar doesn't slide or roll away from you. Place both hands on the opposite end of the bar and raise it to chest height. The bar should be diagonal to your body, pointed away from your torso directly in front of you. Your feet should be shoulder-width apart, knees slightly bent, head up and shoulders back in an athletic stance.

2 In an arcing motion, brace your core and bring the bar to the right side of your body without twisting your hips. Your shoulders should remain in line with your hips, pointed straight ahead as in the start position. Hold this position with your core flexed for 3–5 seconds. Return to start position by swinging the bar in a reverse arc.

3 Repeat to the left side using the opposite motion.

After returning to the top position, bring the bar down toward your waist, pause for 3–5 seconds and press back up to the top position.

Triceps Pressdown

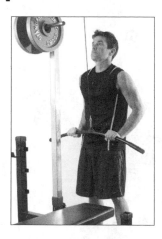

1 Using a triceps pressdown machine or lat pulldown machine, grasp the bar with an overhand grip (palms toward the ground). Pull the bar down until your elbows are aligned with the outside of your body; both will be bent and the bar will be about chin height in front of your body. Engage your core.

2 Keeping your elbows in place, use your triceps (not your shoulders) to pull the bar down in an arc toward your hips. Squeeze your triceps to keep the bar in position, and hold for 1–3 seconds. Do not hunch forward; keep your core engaged and back straight throughout the entire movement.

Slowly return the bar to start position at your chin.

Leg Press

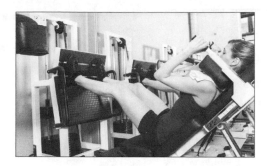

1 Sit in a 45-degree leg press machine. Position your feet so your knees are over your toes. Your feet should be pointed slightly outward and shoulder-width apart.

2 Push through your heels and fully extend your legs.

Pause, then SLOWLY lower the weight to the start position.

Hamstring Curl

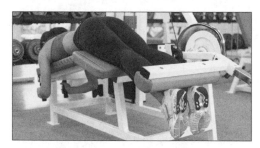

1 Lie face down on a leg curl machine. Position both feet with toes pointing slightly outward.

2 Contract your hamstrings and glutes to bring your heels to your glutes.

Pause, then return to start position.

Basic Jump Rope

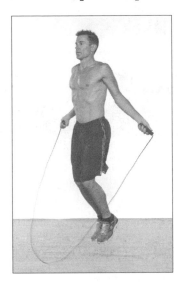

1 Stand erect with your feet approximately shoulder-width apart, knees slightly bent and arms extended along your sides. Throughout the movement your weight should be distributed evenly on the balls of both feet. Grip the jump rope handles using a classic grip. Extend the apex of the jump rope loop on the ground behind your feet.

2 Rotate your wrists forward to swing the rope overhead. The first movement from a dead stop will require more arm and shoulder movement, but as you progress on subsequent jumps, your arms should remain in a semi-static downward position along the sides of your body and your hands should rotate in small arcs.

3 As the apex of the rope's loop approaches the ground in front of your body and is 6 inches away from your toes, jump straight up approximately 4–6 inches off the floor with both feet as the rope passes underneath.

4 Land on the balls of both feet and bend your knees slightly to cushion the impact while continuing to rotate your wrists and swing the rope in an arc from back to front.

Jump Rope: The Skier

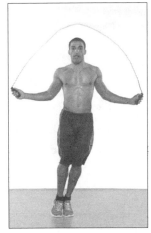 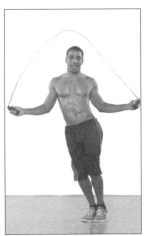

While jumping rope, continuously jump both feet to one side and then the other.

Jump Rope: The Bell

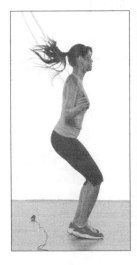 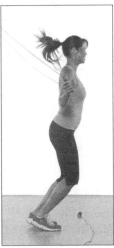

While jumping rope, continuously jump both feet forward and then backward.

Warm-Ups & Stretches

Arm Circle

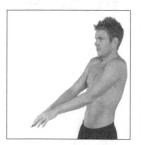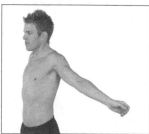

Stand with your feet shoulder-width apart. Move both arms in a complete circle forward 5 times and then backward 5 times.

Chest

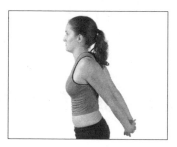

Clasp your hands together behind your lower back with palms facing each other. Keeping an erect posture and your arms as straight as possible, gently pull your arms away from your back, straight out behind you. Keep your shoulders down. Hold for 10 seconds.

Rest for 30 seconds and repeat.

Lower Back

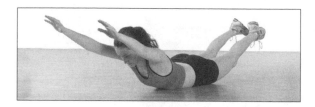

Lying face-down on your stomach, extend your arms along the floor above your head, palms on the ground. Keeping your knees straight, extend your legs behind you, keeping your feet close together and your toes on the ground. In a slow, controlled motion, contract your lower back (erector spinae) and raise your arms and legs 6–8 inches off the floor. Hold for 5 seconds.

Lower slowly back to start position. Repeat slowly 10 times.

Shoulders

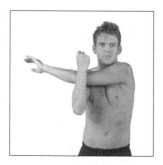

Stand with your feet shoulder-width apart and bring your left arm across your chest. Support your left elbow with the crook of your right arm by raising your right arm to 90 degrees. Gently pull your left arm to your chest while maintaining proper posture (straight back, wide shoulders). Don't round or hunch your shoulders. Hold your arm to your chest for 10 seconds. Release and switch arms.

After you've done both sides, shake your hands out for 5–10 seconds.

Around the World

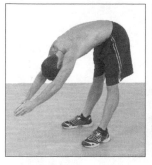 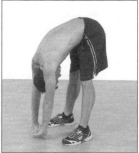

1 Stand with your feet shoulder-width apart and extend your hands overhead with elbows locked, fingers interlocked, and palms up. Keep your arms straight the entire time.

2 Bending at the hips, bring your hands down toward your right leg, and in a continuous circular motion bring your hands toward your toes, then toward your left leg and then return your hands overhead and bend backward.

Repeat three times, then change directions.

"Poor Man's Yoga" Dynamic Warm-Up

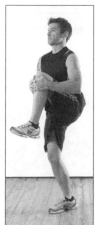 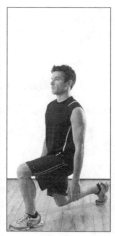 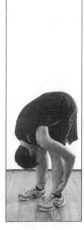

1 Stand up straight in an "athletic stance": shoulders back, head high, back straight, hands at sides, knees

with a slight bend, feet about shoulder-width apart with toes pointed slightly outward. Shift your weight to your right foot while bending your left knee and bringing it up toward your chest. Place your hands on your upper shin, below your knee, and slowly apply force to bring your knee closer to your upper torso while maintaining your balance. Release your left leg if you lose your balance; do not allow your right knee to bow inward or outward as it may result in injury.

2 Slowly, in a controlled manner, release your hands and step forward about 2 feet with your left foot and place it on the ground; drop your hips straight down into a lunge position. Your left leg should be bent 90 degrees, your upper leg parallel with the ground, lower leg perpendicular to it. Your right toes should be on the ground, your right leg bent at 90 degrees as well. Your upper body should be upright, with your head high, shoulders back and core braced to keep your back straight.

3 Slowly press up from your left heel and push your body back into a standing position with both feet parallel. Bend at the waist and bring your head toward your knees, placing your hands on the backs of your lower calves and pulling slightly to assist in getting your noggin closer to your knees. Release your hands and slowly return to the start position. That's 1 rep; repeat with your right leg. Perform 5 reps on each side.

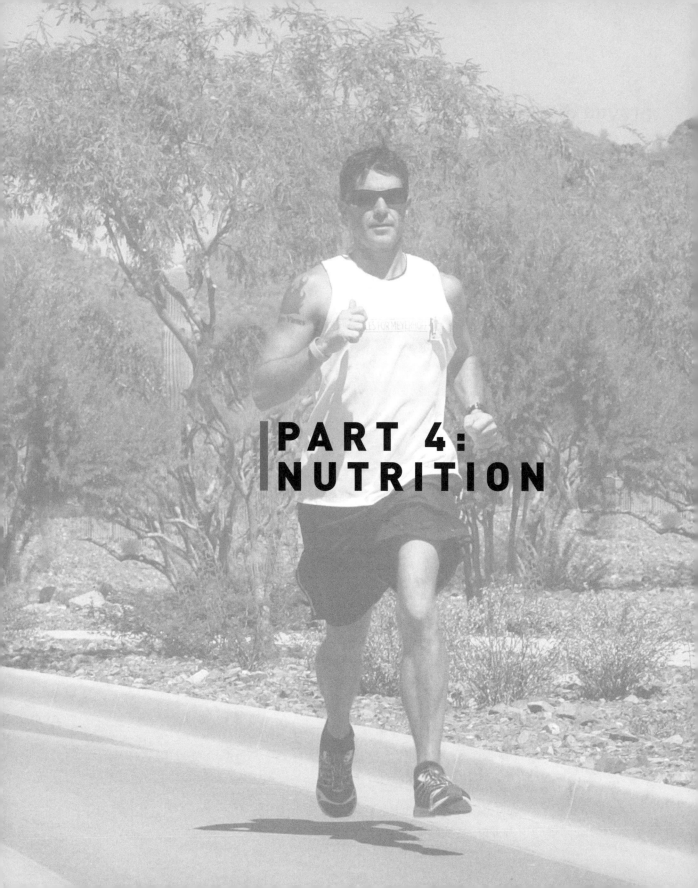

PART 4: NUTRITION

Fueling the Athlete

What's a calorie? Think you know? Nope. Sorry, you're wrong. The term "calories" is really just a convenient, although somewhat inaccurate, way to describe a particular food's effect on your body. Unfortunately, it's too general a term to explain how important different sources of fueling are to your body's performance on a daily basis and in the long run.

Your body actually has no idea what a calorie is—the only thing it understands is that fuel is being added to the system and thousands of different bodily functions are called into action to figure out what to do with it. For instance, 500 pizza calories are treated completely differently from 500 broccoli calories in terms of the way they're processed and utilized.

Just remember, all calories are NOT created equal, but you've surely figured that out by now. "Cutting calories" only works if you're slashing excess ones from your diet (see "How Many Calories Do I Burn?" on page 182) or trimming back the wrong types of calories at the wrong times.

We break the nutrition in this book into three parts. One is geared toward those following the FXT:FIT, FXT:SXP or FXT:EXP programs, where the goal is to get lean, strong and fast and develop long-term athletic endurance. Another is for those following the FXT:MX1 program, who have the very specific goal of gaining muscle as quickly as possible. The third nutrition is for those following FXT:ST1.

There's way too much for us to cover here, so for more resources on calories, nutritional benefits from specific foods and Glycemic Index, visit "Nutrition" on http://fxtfit.com.

Macronutrients Athletes Need

The following is a high-level overview of carbs, fats and proteins to give you a bit of a primer when making your nutritional decisions.

Carbohydrates: Used by the human body as a primary source of energy, carbohydrates are simple or complex sugars that are broken down into glucose within the body. Simple carbohydrates are sugars made of one or two molecules that are easily absorbed into bloodstream and are responsible for rapid, short-term energy boosts. White and brown sugar, honey, corn syrup, jams, jellies and most fruit drinks and soft drinks fall into this category and provide little nutritional benefit other than energy from calories. Most often associated with sweets and candies, simple carbs are often attributed to weight gain from empty calories and a spike in energy followed by a crash of lethargy. For endurance athletes, energy gels and carb-loaded drinks used during extreme training and racing provide a necessary dose of energy during long and grueling events. If an athlete doesn't have the proper amount of glucose, their performance will diminish rapidly as energy stores are depleted, leading to the dreaded "bonk" when their body just runs out of fuel and quits.

To make carbs easier to understand, we classify them into three general groups:

- White Carbs: White bread, pasta, white potatoes and white rice are all examples of simple or complex sugars that have a high glycemic impact that spike your blood sugars quickly for a rapid energy boost, but are torched fairly quickly.

- Brown Carbs: Whole-grain bread, sweet potatoes, quinoa and farro are examples of slower-burning sugars that keep your system fueled for longer periods of time. If white carbs were a match, these would be a candle.

- Green Carbs: Vegetables and fruits provide a mix of fast- and slow-burning carbs from the healthiest of sources. For the most part, fruits provide quick sugars for a pre-

or post-exercise energy boost and veggies provide a slower release of sugars for prolonged energy (not to mention vitamins and minerals to keep your system running at peak performance).

Carbs also play a fundamental role in muscle building. See "The Secret Weapon" on page 177 to learn how to use carbohydrates to your benefit when lifting weights to pack on muscle while following the FXT:MX1 program.

Proteins: Composed of amino acids, this essential nutrient is required by the body for growth and cellular maintenance. Abundant in muscles, protein can be found in all cells of the body and is a major structural component of all organs, hair and skin. The amino acids that provide the building blocks for protein are responsible for building new tissue and repairing damaged tissues, especially muscles. Ingesting protein from food is extremely important, and provides nine essential amino acids that are not synthesized in the body and are vital for building muscle. Lean proteins can be found in chicken, fish, beef, eggs, tofu, milk, yogurt, cheeses and soy-based alternatives. Check the FXT:FIT and FXT:MX1 recommendations on lean protein intake while following each program.

Fats: The "low-fat" diet craze that persisted throughout the end of the twentieth century still has a tiny foothold on some eaters. The thought that fats make you fat and that low-fat foods are better than full-fat items has been completely disproven, yet you'll see plenty of low-fat alternatives if you take a quick peek at any grocery aisle. A quick rule of thumb on low-fat products: Just say no. If you look at the label you'll usually see the fat content is slightly lower and the calories higher—it's not

the fat they take out that's the problem, it's the additional ingredients like sugar that they put in!

Simply put, ingesting fat in moderation does not make you fat. Period. Actually, fat content in food will satiate you for longer periods of time and help prevent cravings to snack in between meals. Monounsaturated and polyunsaturated fats are essential to the human diet as they provide alpha-linolenic acid (omega-3) and linolenic acid (omega-6), which may reduce your risk of sudden cardiac death, lower blood pressure and decrease inflammation, reducing arthritis, decreasing the risk of a heart attack and stroke, reducing depression, preventing dementia, and even reducing the risk of some types of cancer. A very small amount of saturated fat is beneficial for bone and skin health; less than 5% of daily calories are recommended.

Monounsaturated fats are found in olive, canola and sunflower oils, avocados, peanuts, cashews and almonds. Polyunsaturated fats are abundant in flaxseed, safflower oil, walnuts, chia seeds and seaweed. Saturated fats can be found in coconut, palm kernel, cottonseed and chocolate.

All's not completely well in the world of fats, however, as long as trans fats made with hydrogenated or partially hydrogenated oils are in anyone's diet. A 2006 *New England Journal of Medicine* scientific review reported, "From a nutritional standpoint, the consumption of trans fatty acids results in considerable potential harm but no apparent benefit."

Trans fats occur naturally in the meat and milk of cattle and sheep, but the biggest danger comes from hydrogenated or partially hydrogenated oils in any prepared food as they often utilize these potentially harmful trans fats to replace animal fats. Luckily, regulations, bans and various markings on packaging are in place in most Westernized nations around the world, allowing careful consumers to spot and avoid trans fats.

Micronutrients Are a Big Deal

Micronutrients are composed of vitamins and minerals. Your body requires vitamins to regulate its complex chemistry, including that of the digestive and nervous systems. Minerals are the building blocks for bone strength and cardiovascular health.

Meats, fruits and vegetables contain a majority of the vitamins and minerals your body needs on a daily basis, and you're best off getting all your micronutrients from real, whole foods. As an example, red meat contains iron, zinc, phosphorus, niacin, B12, thiamin, riboflavin and vitamin D, while spinach is rich in vitamins A, B2, B6, C, E and K, magnesium, manganese, folate, betaine, iron, calcium, potassium, folic acid, copper, phosphorus, zinc, niacin and selenium. If you're on a restricted diet (e.g., eating fewer than three meals a day and abstaining from certain foods like meat, poultry, fish and dairy), vitamin supplements can be a beneficial way to make sure your body is getting the vital micronutrients it needs.

General Nutrition Tips

Whenever possible, use whole foods instead of powdered supplements or vitamins for your nutritional needs. For instance, the additional fiber from eating a green pepper is preferential to a "green powder" supplement to keep you satiated. That being said, when you're in a hurry, the ability to use a mix or pop a pill makes it easier on the go. There are no perfect mixes of superfoods that contain everything your body needs in one convenient little package—most of it's marketing with a healthy dose of hype. For example, a boring handful of native blueberries contains the same amount of antioxidants or more than the exotic "Amazon superfruit" that costs three or four times as much. A handful of fruits and veggies in a blender is a great start; combine them with a multivitamin and whole foods throughout the day and you're ahead of the game.

As far as deciding what's better or worse for your nutrition when looking at supplements or post-workout recovery drinks, you need to look at the labels and consider what fits your goals best. If you're keeping carbs or calories low or shooting for a specific target number of protein grams, then choose accordingly. The bottom line is, do some homework and remember this mantra: "No matter what the front of the label says, the only thing that really matters is what the back of the label says in the Nutritional Information section."

Always read the small print on labels just like you would when signing a legal agreement. Consider the stuff you put in your body just as important as any other contract you'd sign.

The "best" fueling and nutrition is entirely subjective since everyone's complex system works differently. It requires a lot of introspection and testing to figure out what works best for you. Anyone who tells you something is the best for you is a liar—it may be perfect for them while being suboptimal for you. We've trained with football linebackers who drink two gallons of milk a day and marathoners who gorge on pizza and beer every Saturday. Neither approach may be ideal for you, but it works for them.

Start with lean proteins, healthy fats and slow-burning (brown or green) carbs and then build your daily and weekly intake from there. Once you get that down, tweak it for certain situations, such as eating fast-burning carbs during a long-distance event or 15 minutes before a high-intensity workout.

The Bottom Line: Eat healthy, lean meats, fresh fruit and vegetables while limiting processed foods and sugars. As a baseline, follow the Institute of Medicine's recommendation and get up to 35% of your daily calories from lean proteins, 45% from high-quality carbs and 20% from healthy fats. It's really not hard to follow, and the results will be noticeable.

Nutrition for FXT:FIT, FXT:SXP & FXT:EXP

In order to build a lean physique and keep your energy level high enough for the intensity of the Fit, Speed and Endurance workouts, you need to get enough macro- and micronutrients and hydration. This is a pretty generic statement since the only way you'll figure out your exact nutritional needs is through trial and error. Below are some guidelines, and each of the workout programs also contains some specific tips as well.

The FXT:FIT, FXT:SXP and FXT:EXP are progressively more difficult and demanding from a fueling and meal-timing standpoint, so you'll need to closely monitor your performance in order to dial in a mean schedule that works for you. Some athletes choose to distribute their nutrition into six small meals by eating every two hours throughout the day. This helps to keep certain athletes feeling satiated and their energy reserves topped off all day long, but it's not necessarily the end-all, be-all of daily nutritional intake. We've worked with some athletes who base their daily meals around several healthy snacks and one big feast midday, and others who subscribe to the standard three-meals-a-day regimen. All are successful in their own way, and as long as it provides the necessary energy for training, racing, recovery and rebuilding for each athlete, then it's the "right one" for them!

You'll need to do a little bit of trial and error to fit your specific fueling needs as you increase your training intensity, and even retool it as you move on to FXT:SXP and FXT:EXP. With the progressively increasing demands in each successive program, you'll most likely have to increase your total caloric intake for your pre- and post-workout meals.

A mix of slow- and fast-burning carbs such as steel-cut oatmeal with cinnamon, wheat toast with a little bit of peanut butter and half a banana are good examples of a quick meal in the morning before a workout. The latter even includes some protein to aid in muscle recovery.

Consuming a recovery drink after a hard workout that has a 4:1 ratio of fast-burning carbs to protein. An 8- to 10-ounce glass of chocolate milk or recovery sports drink can do the trick.

Include some lean proteins in every meal— shoot for .55–1 gram of protein per pound of body weight. A 150-pound athlete would require between 82.5 and 150 grams of protein per day.

Eat healthily, eat often. If you're eating fresh, whole foods, specifically vegetables, fruits, lean proteins, slow-burning carbs and some healthy fats, you shouldn't really have to worry about your calorie and macro-/micronutrient intake while you're progressing through the programs—you'll pretty much have it covered. If you're feeling weak and lethargic, try increasing pre- and post-workout carbs a little bit. If you feel bloated, trim back white carbs a bit.

Eat lightly before a run or hard workout. This goes without saying, but it's oft-forgotten— don't try and run or workout at high intensity with too many solids in your stomach, as your body will divert blood flow to your muscles and leave your stomach feeling queasy.

Nutrition for Building Muscle & Developing Strength

If you want to sculpt your physique and pack on the muscle, you must start in the kitchen. Eating right is 80% of the battle right there. Sure, you have to strength train to get and stay buff, which is the other very crucial 20% percent, but you also have to actively pay attention to what you're putting into your mouth and stay in control of your choices. After all, you and you alone are responsible for deciding what you eat. The keys to success in this regard are simple: remain aware of your food intake and plan out your meals in advance. Toward that end, we'll be providing tips to help you accomplish both.

In order to pack on muscle, you'll need to change two major aspects of your eating: first, up your total weekly caloric intake (most people will have to up the total caloric intake of all three macros: fat, protein and carbs). The second thing you'll need to change, and by far the most important, is the amount and timing of those macros. There's a secret to gaining muscle, and that's our secret weapon.

FXT:MX1 Basic Nutrition Principles

At this point we've talked about the necessity of lifting heavy weights to build muscle. But lifting alone won't cut it! If all we did was lift heavy weights, we would've essentially primed the body for growth but, without changing our diet, we won't be fueling it to grow. So, with that, we need to talk about our basic food and eating principles.

These principles are the basis for FXT:MX1, and understanding them will allow you to adjust and adapt the programs to suit your needs and body. For the vast majority of people, the principles for both muscle and strength are going to be the same. The total number of calories, macro ratios and number of carbs might differ, but the principles are the same. People looking to build muscle should pay closer attention to the mirror everyday and those looking for strength, while noting their appearance in the mirror, should watch the numbers on the bar and how they feel both working out and recovering.

THE SECRET WEAPON

Want to gain muscle? Want to get bigger? Want to dramatically change your appearance? There are two things you need in your arsenal: heavy weights and carbohydrates (a.k.a. carbs). We've already talked about the heavy weights—now we're going to talk about the carbs.

Carbs, specifically carb timing, is the single most important thing to nailing in your diet as you fight to gain muscle. Simply put: no carbs before a workout (#3), carbs with protein after a workout (#4), and minimal carbs on non-workout days (#5).

The second secret to carbs is carb-cycling: alternating days of high and low carbs depending on your activity level. This is an incredibly old-school bodybuilding technique to gain lean muscle while keeping fat gain to an absolute minimum. This technique has been revamped in many modern approaches and we'll expose what we've found to be the most effective.

Here are seven principles to follow when you're looking to build muscle.

1. SKIP BREAKFAST.

Frankly, breakfast sucks. It's overrated and has many detrimental effects on the body, including cutting into the fat-burning window and priming your body for fat storage. If you MUST eat breakfast, a high-protein, zero-carb, moderate-/low-fat breakfast is best. We don't recommend breakfast to anyone except the hardest of gainers and, frankly, even they should skip it.

Why? When you wake up your body is at the highest point of insulin sensitivity for the entire day. If you did nothing different during the day, your body will slowly become more insulin insensitive as the day progresses. That's why we recommend you skip breakfast. Eating food, specifically carbs, and to a lesser degree fat, when you're insulin sensitive is a great way to gain fat. And that's actually what the general breakfast case is—a great way to gain fat.

2. THE LATER IN THE DAY YOU WORK OUT, THE BETTER.

We've found this to be the hardest to implement in practice, but it has the most upside. The later in the day you work out, the more food options you have and the better your gains will be. The optimal time to work out would be any time past 4 p.m. (assuming normal sleeping patterns). If you can work out later in the day, you can get away with eating more fun foods than you can earlier in the day. The more extreme version is working out first thing in the morning. Sorry to say, but your options are limited here.

Why? As we said in the breakfast section, as the day progresses your body becomes less sensitive to insulin spikes, meaning it becomes harder to store food as fat. Working out later in the day primes your body to build muscle. And by fueling with carbs and protein, your body will be packing on solid slabs of muscle and minimal or no fat.

3. CONSUME ONLY PROTEIN AND FAT BEFORE A WORKOUT.

Assuming for the sake of argument you work out after 5 p.m., eat only protein and fat before your workout, and limit the total caloric intake to roughly 30% of your total for the day. This might be rough for some people, but you want to save your calories for when your body is going to use them the most: post-workout. The reason to only eat protein and fat and not carbs is that you haven't primed your body to use the carbs yet; you haven't worked out.

Why? Special things happen when you lift heavy weights, but when you haven't lifted yet, you can't take advantage of them. In essence, the body isn't ready to take advantage of carbs,

and by feeding carbs when the body isn't ready makes it much more likely those carbs will be stored as fat, not muscle. You still need to fuel the body to build muscle and the way you achieve this is through fats and proteins.

4. CONSUME ONLY PROTEIN AND CARBS AFTER A WORKOUT.

After a workout your body is ready to grow. You've stimulated the body, putting it in a position to soak up nutrients and repair the muscle fibers. Now's the time to feed it! Protein helps grow and build the muscles while carbs shuttle protein to the muscles. It's as simple as that.

Why? Now you're ready to build muscle and you want to fuel that. Carbs are the mechanism to spike insulin levels to shuttle the protein to the muscles.

5. NO WORKOUT? NO CARBS.

This is an easy rule to follow and you can immediately see the application. If you don't work out very hard with heavy weights, don't even think about eating carbs. Non-workout days? Fats and protein, baby! Before you work out in the day? Yeah, same answer—all fats and protein.

Why? Carbs are for post-workout when you've primed your body to grow. If you haven't worked out yet or you're on an off day, you haven't stressed your body, therefore it can't and won't use the carbs to grow muscle. Why would you give it carbs then? If you wanted to gain fat, that would be a perfect time to eat carbs, but since that isn't your goal, no carbs.

6. TYPE IS OVERRATED.

Clean foods, organic sources, grass-fed, non-farmed, etc.—it gets confusing and, we're happy to say, is completely overrated. It's far more important to nail your macro levels and the timing of the food rather than the type of food. We have a saying: "First optimize what food you eat, then optimize what food your food eats."

Caveat: The one and only caveat with the above is the type of carb you eat. There's one time during the day the type of carb matters: Post-workout you want high-GI carbs (think dextrose, white rice, white potato). The sooner you spike your insulin and get your body rebuilding muscle, the better. Our recommended post-workout shake has whey protein isolate, creatine, leucine and dextrose— all the things a growing body needs! You can check out some of our favorite muscle-building shake recipes on www.fxtfit.com/nutrition.

7. KEEP AN EATING WINDOW.

One of the early mistakes Jason made was having too big a carb window, meaning he worked out too early in the day and freely ate carbs until he went to sleep. There are two ways to keep a window: work out later in the day so your natural window is between your workout and bed or to still workout earlier, say noon, and eat your carbs for only a two-hour or so window. The approach you take is up to you. You'll need to watch how your body reacts and adjust accordingly. We strongly recommend you work out later in the day to have a natural window between the workout and going to bed.

FXT:ST1 Basic Nutrition Principles

The overlap between muscle and strength nutrition is high, but there are more tweaks that can be made when the goal is developing strength. The key is to understand your body and how you respond. Most people can and should use the FXT:MX1 nutrition principles

laid out earlier in this chapter. However, some people will need to tweak those principles. Those tweaks are laid out below.

TWEAK #1. FUEL THE WORKOUT WITH CARBS.

Some people find that not having carbs in their system before a workout makes getting through the strength workouts a real challenge. There are several approaches that work well here; just make sure you pay close attention to what works best for you.

APPROACH 1: PRE-WORKOUT NUTRITION

Most people could and should follow the guidelines on page 178 and only consume fat and protein before a workout. However, if your workouts are suffering and you feel you need a bit extra, before a workout have a small meal of protein and carbs, probably 20–30 grams of each, about an hour or so before your workout. You don't need to go nuts here— just enough to fuel the workout.

Have a drink or some carbs handy during your workout and slowly drink or eat that throughout the workout. A sugary drink (not soda!) or a banana works well.

After your workout, a little dextrose in your protein shake would be fine. After that, go straight back to just protein and fat.

APPROACH 2: CARB UP THE NIGHT BEFORE A WORKOUT

This approach is more aggressive and basically moves the post-workout carb load to the night before. The idea is to fill up your glucose reserves for the workout the next day. You can have some fun here; just don't go too crazy. The idea is to consume just enough carbs to get you through the workout the next day. You'll have to play around and understand how much you need. Start on the lower side of the amount of carbs you'll need and see how it goes.

TWEAK #2. CONSUME CARBS EVERY DAY.

This is the most aggressive version and should be used only in extreme cases. This isn't for most people and should be used primarily by those who are very underweight or particularly weak.

APPROACH 1: PRIMARY CARB LOAD THE DAY BEFORE WORKOUT

This is the same as loading up on carbs the night before a workout, except you'll also eat carbs the night of a workout. The difference is in the amounts. Consume your normal amount the day before and about half that amount the day of the workout.

APPROACH 2: PRIMARY CARB LOAD THE DAY OF WORKOUT

This is exactly the opposite of Approach #1. You'll consume your goal carbs the day of the workout after your workout, mostly at night, and about half that amount the night before your workout.

APPROACH 3: CARBS ALL THE TIME

The single most-aggressive approach has you consuming the same number of carbs the night before and the night of your workout. Using this approach it's very easy to go overboard and put on fat just as easily as putting on muscle. Pay attention, be careful and know your goals.

APPENDIX

Weight Loss: The First Step on Your Fitness Journey

Back on page 169 we talked a little bit about calories and why they're so important for athletes. Here we give you the calculations to help you decide how many calories you need to take in on a daily basis to keep up with your body's needs. You can use the BMI formula to assess your body mass index, figure out where you are on the scale and adjust your goals and workouts accordingly.

WHAT'S MY BODY MASS INDEX (BMI)?

It's necessary to assess your body mass index, or BMI, in order to somewhat better understand what your plan of action should be to healthily start slimming down. (*Note:* BMI does not account for muscle mass, so is relatively inaccurate in assessing muscular individuals, usually putting them incorrectly in the "obese" category.)

The BMI formula is a little complicated:

WEIGHT (IN POUNDS) /
[HEIGHT (IN INCHES)]^2
X 703

Calculate BMI by dividing weight in pounds by height in inches squared and multiplying by a conversion factor of 703.

Example:

Weight = 150 pounds
Height = 65" (5'5")

Calculation:
[150 ÷ (65)^2] x 703 = 24.96

(The U.S. Center for Disease Control provides an easy calculator online: http://www.cdc.gov/healthyweight/assessing/ bmi.)

If you're obese and sedentary (BMI higher than 25), you can drop 1–3 pounds per week by adding 20 minutes of exercise (as little as walking or some simple calisthenics) to your regimen each day. Don't make any drastic changes to your nutrition at the same time. Take 2–3 weeks and focus on adding 20 minutes of exercise to your daily routine before adding in some of the meal timings and nutritional suggestions noted on page 174.

For those in the "normal" rating of BMI (18.5–24.9), you can see some positive results by adding 20 minutes of exercise if you're normally sedentary, and will see enhanced results by eating healthier food choices—more vegetables; leaner, higher-protein meats; fewer processed carbohydrates; fewer snacks and fried foods. You can also limit your caloric intake as much as 500 calories below your BMR (see page 183).

If you're below 18.5 on the BMI scale, you'll actually need to take in more calories while adding a running and cross-training regimen to your routine. Adding 200 to 500 calories in vegetables, lean meats, healthy fats (nuts, oils, avocados) and non-processed carbs will help you stay lean while also giving your body the fuel it needs to perform well under the new demands of a training routine.

HOW MANY CALORIES DO I BURN?

Here's a little cheat sheet to give you an idea what your calorie burn is really like so you can think twice before "treating yourself" to a celebratory doughnut after your workout. Calculations are based on the amount of calories a 150-pound man can expect to burn in 1 hour:

Walking at 19:00 pace: ~230 calories
Running at 10:00 pace: ~700 calories
Sitting on couch: ~100 calories

The last one may throw you for a loop. You would've burned about 100 calories by sitting on your butt and letting your body's systems do their thing. Your BMR, or basal metabolic rate, is essentially the amount of calories your body would burn if you stayed in bed all day long, and it's probably higher than you think. Simply stated, the BMR is the base (basal) amount of energy (calories, nutrients) needed for your body to function (metabolic rate). The good news: Twenty-four hours a day, your body burns calories to keep going, whether or not you're exercising. The not-necessarily-breaking news: In the example above, the 150-pound man walking at a 19:00 pace for an hour burned an additional 130 calories versus just sitting on the couch (230 by walking –100 BMR). Don't worry, even those 130 calories add up: Over one month of walking for one hour daily would result in burning around an additional pound of body fat versus sitting on the couch. Jogging at 10:00 pace, the fat burn would be over 4.5 pounds!

BMR Formula for men:

BMR = 66 + (6.23 X WEIGHT IN POUNDS)

+ (12.7 X HEIGHT IN INCHES)

- (6.8 X AGE IN YEARS)

For example, Brett is 5'9" (69"), 155 pounds and 42 years of age; his BMR is 1622.35.

BMR Formula for women:

BMR = 65

+ (4.35 X WEIGHT IN POUNDS)

+ (4.7 X HEIGHT IN INCHES)

- (4.7 X AGE IN YEARS)

HOW MANY CALORIES DO I NEED?

Once you know how many calories your body requires just to keep functioning, you need to calculate your daily output (work, play, exercise) requirements to keep your system fueled with the energy it needs. Based on your daily level of activity, multiply your BMR by the factor in the table below to get the number of calories you should consume in a day to maintain your weight and proper bodily functions.

CALORIC INTAKE (HARRIS BENEDICT FORMULA)

Sedentary, little or no exercise:
BMR x 1.2

Light exercise or sports 1–3 days per week:
BMR x 1.375

Moderate exercise or sports 3–5 days per week:
BMR x 1.55

Hard exercise or sports 6–7 days per week:
BMR x 1.725

Very hard exercise, amateur to professional athlete:
BMR x 1.9

For instance, with Brett's BMR of 1622.35 and a multiplier of 1.725 during hard training, his caloric intake should be around 2800 calories per day.

If you're planning to use this BMR and caloric intake chart to lose weight, don't go overboard. Reducing your intake by 500 calories a day is a substantial amount and a good guideline to go by for healthy weight loss when combined with light to moderate exercise. If you plan on upping the intensity, keep your calories right around the calculated number above and you should lose weight effectively as well.

Nutrition plays a big part in fueling for training and getting the long-term body composition you want. Refer to "Fueling the Athlete" on page 169 for guidelines on macro- and micronutrient consumption. You'll also learn about how what you take in before, during and after training affects your success.

Additional Exercises

Here are some other great full-body exercises to add to your workout.

ROPE CLIMB

INITIAL HAND PLACEMENT: Jump and extend your arms to reach and grasp the rope as high as you can with both hands, one above the other. Steady yourself on the rope while you prepare to get your feet into the position of your choice.

FOOT PLACEMENT—PINCH METHOD: This is the best method for climbing a rope with knots; you'll pinch your feet together above the knot and "stand" on it while you reach up and reposition your hands. When climbing a rope without knots, this method is greatly dependent on the strength of your leg adductor muscles and the grip on the instep of your footwear to keep your feet locked in place on the rope. This is the most inefficient way to climb a knotless

rope, resulting in wasted energy and worn-out arms, core, and legs as your feet invariably slip down the rope.

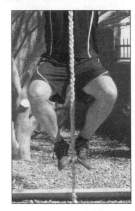

HOW TO DO IT: With your arms extended overhead and hands holding the rope tightly, squeeze both of your feet together loosely with the rope between the insteps of both feet, and bend at your waist to raise your legs as close to your hands as possible. Squeeze your feet together tightly (preferably on top of a knot) to hold your place on the rope while you extend your torso, "stand up" and reach your hands up as high as possible on the rope. Repeat until you get to the top. Use the pinching to slow your descent, lowering your hands one under the other until your feet are safely on the ground. Do not slide down the rope!

FOOT PLACEMENT—CALF WRAP METHOD: This is commonly known as the "Marine Brake and Squat" and is much more efficient than the pinch method because the rope is held securely by wrapping it around your calf and then looping it under one and over the other foot. Famous for rope burns, this method is best accomplished while wearing long pants or tall socks.

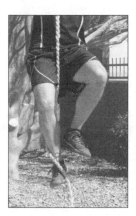

HOW TO DO IT: With your arms extended overhead and hands gripping the rope, allow the rope to hang between your legs. Rotate your right leg clockwise (counter-clockwise with your left leg if you prefer) around the rope so that it wraps around your lower leg and then the outside of your right foot. Take your left foot and loop it under the rope so that the rope is under your right foot and on top of your left. Pressing your left foot on top of your right foot to trap the rope between them acts as a brake to lock the rope in place. Release the tension between your feet and allow the rope to slide around your leg as you squat and raise your feet upward toward your hands. Clamp your left foot on top of your right to secure your foot position while you stand up and reach as high as you can to get a new grip on the rope. Repeat all the way until you reach the top of the rope. Use the foot brake to slow your descent, lowering your hands one under the other until your feet are safely on the ground. Do not slide down the rope!

FOOT PLACEMENT—TACTICAL SPEED CLIMB: This is undoubtedly the fastest way to climb a rope while using your feet (arm-only is the fastest altogether) and has the added benefit of not resulting in as many rope burns and can be performed rather comfortably in shorts. Perfected and used by military Special Operations personnel, this method is the most efficient.

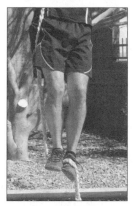

HOW TO DO IT: With your arms extended overhead and hands holding the rope, allow the rope to fall to the outside of your right leg (swap the directions for opposite legs if you prefer). Loop your left foot under the rope so that it's under your right foot and on top of your left. Press your left foot on top of your right foot and trap the rope between them to lock the rope in place. Release the tension between your feet and allow it to slide around your leg as you squat and raise your feet upward toward your hands. Clamp your left foot on top of your right to secure your foot position while you stand up and reach as high as you can to get a new grip on the rope. Repeat all the way until you reach the top of the rope. Use the foot brake to slow your descent, lowering your hands one under the other until your feet are safely on the ground. Do not slide down the rope!

FXT:Travel: 10-Minute Workout

Quite possibly the easiest program in the world to remember, this 10-minute workout alternates between up and down moves to work your entire body. Whether you've jogged to a park while on vacation or are stuck in a hotel room killing time before the big meeting (plan time for a shower, OK?), you can follow this daily routine to get in a simple workout on the road to keep the blood flowing and your workouts on track. Consider this your "no excuse" program, as in you have absolutely no excuse for not performing a quick 10-minute set like this 3–5 times a week, no matter where in the world you find yourself. It only takes a tiny investment of time and pays dividends in your health and fitness. Unlike any of the other programs, there are no target points or target time—this is a quick, simple, no-fail program.

- 10 Toe Touches (each foot) *page 151*

- 10 Marching Twists (each leg) *page 142*

- 20 Jumping Jacks *page 142*

- 10 Push-Ups *page 156*

- 10 Sit-Ups *page 138*

- 20 Squats *page 148*

- 10 Chair Dips *page 160*

That's it, you're done! (If you have a little more time and feel good, do another round.) In order to keep fit and active, you can use a simple program like this one to bridge the gap between workouts when you're extremely busy, traveling or just getting back into exercising after some time off. For a more advanced program, check out Intro to FXT:PX1 on page 71 to really get back in the swing!

Index

Photo Credits

page 5: © Scott E. Whitney

page 20: © Scott E. Whitney

page 23: © photobank.kiev.ua/shutterstock.com

page 45: © Rapt Productions

page 47: © Scott E. Whitney

page 130: © Scott E. Whitney

page 131: © Rapt Productions

page 132: V-Sit © Rapt Productions; Ab Crunch with Toe Touch © Scott E. Whitney

page 133: Mason Twist © Rapt Productions; T-Twist © Scott E. Whitney

page 134: Elephant Twist © Scott E. Whitney; Wood Chop and Flutter Kick © Rapt Productions

page 135: © Scott E. Whitney

page 136: Plank © Rapt Productions; Roll-Out © Scott E. Whitney

page 137: © Rapt Productions

page 138: Sit-Up © Scott E. Whitney; Crunch and Bicycle Crunch © Rapt Productions

page 139: Reverse Crunch © Rapt Productions; Plank Row and Side Plank Fly © Scott E. Whitney

page 140: T Push-Up © Scott E. Whitney; Stability Ball Extension © Rapt Productions

page 141: Hip Raise and Hanging Leg Raise © Rapt Productions; Weighted Hip Thrust © Scott E. Whitney

page 142: © Rapt Productions

page 143: Skater Hop © Scott E. Whitney; Side Hop © Rapt Productions

page 144: © Rapt Productions

page 145: © Scott E. Whitney

page 146: © Scott E. Whitney

page 147: © Scott E. Whitney

page 148: Squat © Rapt Productions; Goblet Squat and Back Squat © Scott E. Whitney

page 149: © Scott E. Whitney

page 150: Lunge © Rapt Productions; Jump Lunge © Scott E. Whitney

page 151: Lunge with Twist © Rapt Productions; Toe Touch © Brett Stewart

page 152: © Scott E. Whitney

page 153: © Scott E. Whitney

page 154: Calf Raise © Scott E. Whitney; Linear Reactive Step-Up © Kristen Stewart

page 155: Step-Up with Dumbbell Curl © Scott E. Whitney; Box Jump © Kristen Stewart

page 156: © Rapt Productions

page 157: Chin-Up © Rapt Productions; Single-Arm Curl & Overhead Press and Overhead Press © Scott E. Whitney

page 158: © Scott E. Whitney

page 159: © Scott E. Whitney

page 160: © Scott E. Whitney

page 161: © Scott E. Whitney

page 162: © Scott E. Whitney

page 163: © Scott E. Whitney

page 164: Triceps Pressdown © Scott E. Whitney; Leg Press © Minerva Studio/shutterstock.com; Hamstring Curl © Philip Date/shutterstock.com

page 165: © Rapt Productions

page 166: © Rapt Productions

page 167: Around the World © Rapt Productions; "Poor Man's Yoga" Dynamic Warm-Up © Scott E. Whitney

page 168: © Michael Bennett

page 184: © Kristen Stewart

page 185: © Kristen Stewart

page 192: © Scott E. Whitney

About the Authors

Brett Stewart is a certified personal trainer, a running and triathlon coach, and an endurance athlete who currently resides in Phoenix, Arizona. An avid multisport athlete, Brett has competed in well over a hundred events, including road races, triathlons, marathons, ultramarathons and OCRs. He's constantly looking for new fitness challenges and developing new workouts and routines for himself, his friends and his clients. Brett can be contacted at www.7weekstofitness.com and is available for speaking at corporate wellness and fitness events across the United States.

Jason Warner is an ISSA Certified Strength Trainer, fitness and sports enthusiast, ultra-marathoner, triathlete, CrossFitter and overall Olympic-lifting nut. He recently relocated to Victoria, British Columbia, from Adelaide, South Australia, with his wife and three young children. Jason wrote *Ultimate Jump Rope Workouts* and *7 Weeks to 10 Pounds of Muscle*, and contributed heavily to *7 Weeks to 50 Pull-Ups* and *7 Weeks to Getting Ripped*.

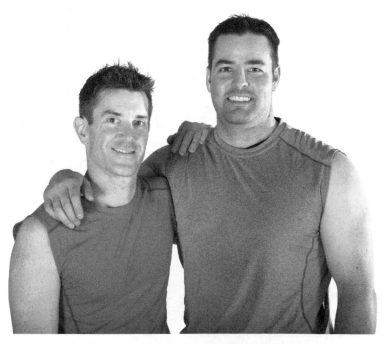

Authors Brett Stewart and Jason Warner